A Practical Guide to Healthy Aging

A Practical Guide to Healthy Aging:

Strategies to Achieve Physical and Mental Health

Andrea Jo Rodgers, PT, DPT, CLT-LANA
Doctor of Physical Therapy

A Practical Guide to Healthy Aging: Strategies to Achieve Physical and Mental Health

Disclaimer

Dedication

This book is dedicated to all my physical therapy outpatients, past, present, and future. It has been an honor and pleasure to work with each and every one of you. I hope you remain on the path to healthy aging!

Table of Contents

Introduction

*C*lint Edwards pauses to catch his breath as he walks along a gently sloped gravel driveway towards his mailbox. "How did I get so old?" he wonders. He recalls a time when he was a star athlete on his high school track team. Nowadays, he tires so easily he isn't sure if he'll be able to go on a once-in-a-lifetime Alaskan cruise this summer with his family. It isn't just his lungs that are giving him a problem. His back is sore and achy, which makes it difficult to sleep. His orthopedic doctor told him he has bone-on-bone arthritis in his right knee, and he should seriously consider getting a total joint replacement. Over the years, his blood pressure has crept up as a "spare tire" permanently settled around his waist. He doesn't even want to step on a scale anymore. This isn't how he'd envisioned his retirement years.

Aging can be defined as the process of growing old. The key to graceful aging is to stay in good health as the years slip by. One of the best ways to do this is to be proactive. What you do today can help ensure better health tomorrow.

People often start to think about aging when something goes amiss. Perhaps they develop an ache or pain that lingers: a stiff neck, an achy back, or painful hips and knees. They may receive a diagnosis that forces them to confront their health head-on, such as hypertension (high blood pressure), high cholesterol, obesity, or perhaps even cancer.

I've worked as a clinical Doctor of Physical Therapy in both the hospital and outpatient setting for thirty years. During this time, I've helped people with wellness initiatives as well as various health problems. I'm CAPP-certified in pelvic health by the American Physical Therapy Association, a nationally certified lymphedema therapist, a PORi-certified oncology rehabilitation therapist, and a certified low pressure fitness instructor. During my 38 years as a volunteer emergency medical technician (EMT) with my local rescue squad, I've assisted countless people in times of medical crisis. The goal of this book is to share pearls of wisdom that I've learned from my experiences as a physical therapist and EMT.

Some may be reading this book to stay healthy as you get older. Others may be looking for ideas to improve your current condition. Perhaps you are looking to build muscle and bone strength, improve flexibility, or choose a healthier lifestyle with respect to diet and exercise. Or maybe you wish to stop leaking urine or say goodbye to constipation and countless hours in the bathroom.

Do you think wellness simply means freedom from disease? Well, it includes much more than that. Wellness can be defined as the state of being in good health, especially as an actively pursued goal. Wellness serves as a cornerstone towards the vision of healthy aging.

Wellness constitutes a dynamic process of change and growth in which individuals actively become aware of healthy choices and consciously make a decision to choose them. It's a balanced lifestyle which encourages physical and mental health and well-being. Wellness emphasizes the mind, body, and spirit.

Emotional wellness allows us to explore our feelings as we cope with life's challenges. Physical wellness involves annual check-ups with your physician, screening for colon cancer as recommended by your doctor, and getting an annual mammogram. Getting your vision and hearing checked, dental visits, choosing to eat a nutritional diet, and exercise are examples of physical wellbeing. Wellness also includes social aspects such as our ability to engage in meaningful relationships with family, friends, and co-workers. Improving cognitive wellness entails embracing lifelong learning. We can enhance our intellectual wellness by seeking out challenges and being open to new concepts and ideas. Learning new skills helps us make personal decisions as we negotiate the curveballs life throws at us. Spiritual wellness focuses on our ability to find peace and be in harmony with the world around us. For some, religious faith plays a prominent role in achieving spiritual wellness.

Wellness means being proactive about staying healthy as you get older. It involves using available knowledge and tools to achieve optimal health. Many of the chapters in this book focus on different areas of wellness as a means to strive towards healthy aging. My goal is that each of you stay active, embark on a journey of wellness, and enjoy your middle age and golden years in good mental, physical, emotional, and spiritual health. I hope reading this book will set you on a path towards healthy aging.

Part I: A Practical Guide to Vascular Health

Chapter 1

Use It or Lose It

*T*ina *rejoices at finally being home after a bout of viral pneumonia that landed her in a hospital bed for two weeks. She is shocked at how much the muscles in her legs have shrunk in such a short period of time. Just climbing the stairs to the second floor of her home feels like she is scaling Mount Everest. Have her legs literally turned into toothpicks?*

Who wants to lose their independence and become dependent on others for assistance? Probably not too many. Deconditioning, which is a loss of physical fitness and a deterioration of heart and skeletal muscle due to being sedentary, can put you at risk. Just ten days of bedrest, or complete inactivity, can cause you to lose two pounds of leg muscle![1] Older adults on bedrest tend to lose muscle mass more quickly than their younger counterparts. This is particularly the case for frail, elderly people who are unable to reposition themselves in bed. Moreover, muscles and connective tissue can shorten, leading to contractures of the joints. Bedrest also leads to a decrease in bone density, placing people at risk for osteoporosis (more about osteoporosis in Chapter 12).

"Use it or lose it." If you don't use your muscles, they start to atrophy (get smaller and weaker). In contrast, being physically active may delay the effects of aging and improve your health.[2] People are living longer and longer. According to the Centers for Disease Control and Prevention (CDC), the average life expectancy at birth for the entire United States population was 78.6 years in 2016 (76.1 years for men and 81.1 years for women). The key is to retain independence as you get older. Wouldn't you like to enjoy a vibrant, active lifestyle dining out with family and friends, shopping, and even traveling in your golden years?

Exercise offers a host of benefits. It helps maintain and increase bone mineral density. If you fall, dense bones are less likely to fracture. Exercise increases muscle mass and strength, which improves your balance and helps you stay active and independent. It also lowers blood sugar. Aerobic exercise decreases blood pressure in people with normal blood pressure as well as in those who are hypertensive.[3] Exercise increases HDL (good cholesterol) and decreases triglycerides (fat in the blood).[4,5] In addition, research indicates that people who are active may have less cognitive decline as they age than people who are sedentary.

Performing stretches to improve flexibility is an important component to healthy aging. As people get older, joints may get stiffer and muscles tighter. We need flexibility to fully use our joints when we perform activities of daily living such as dressing, bending, lifting, and reaching. Performing a few simple stretches each day will go a long way in preserving joint mobility. Sometimes, stretching is enough to relieve pain caused by tightness. In Part III: Keeping Your Framework Healthy--A Guide to Healthy Muscles, Joints, and Bones, we'll look in detail at ways to improve your musculoskeletal system.

The idea of "use it or lose it" doesn't just apply to skeletal muscle strength and flexibility, but cardiovascular health as well. The chapters in Part I of this book will provide specific details about cardiovascular exercise. Ideally, choose an aerobic activity that you enjoy, such as walking, cycling, or swimming. For example, you can invest in your future health by buying a pair of sneakers and starting a walking program. If you live in an area that's very hot or cold, try going to a gym or investing in a treadmill or stationary bike for your home. The activity should be performed vigorously enough to raise your heart rate. To achieve and maintain optimal cardiovascular health, aim to exercise for 30 minutes four to five times a week.

Lastly, the concept of "use it or lose it" applies not just to our physical bodies, but our minds as well. Just like your body, your brain performs better if you use it regularly. We'll explore this concept in detail in Part V: Wellness: Healthy Body, Spirit, and Mind.

Chapter 2

Goodbye Couch Potato: Aerobic Activity for Heart Health

Jerry Brown flips through a bunch of television channels as he munches on potato chips and washes them down with crisp lemon-lime soda. Deep down, he knows he should get off his butt and move around. His waistline is expanding weekly. He decides tomorrow will be different. He is going to start taking a walk every day. Maybe even join a gym. He knows it's time for a change. He feels like being a couch potato is going to put him into an early grave.

Why wait until tomorrow? He pushes the bag of potato chips aside. With a heave, he struggles to his feet and shuffles toward the front door. He decides he'll start by walking one block out and one block back and build up gradually from there.

Aerobic means occurring in the presence of oxygen. Sometimes aerobic exercise is referred to as "cardio" because it improves cardiorespiratory fitness. When you perform an aerobic activity, you'll breathe faster and more deeply in response to repeatedly moving the large muscles in your arms and legs. This increase in your respiratory (breathing) rate maximizes the amount of oxygen in your blood. Your heartbeat increases, providing more blood flow to your muscles and lungs. In response, your capillaries (small blood vessels) dilate to deliver more oxygen to your muscles. At the same time, the capillaries carry away waste products, such as carbon dioxide and lactic acid.

Let's pretend you begin a brisk walk (moderate intensity). As you breathe in, oxygen enters your lungs, is processed, and is then sent via your blood vessels to your heart. The heart pumps the oxygen-rich blood via your arteries to your entire body, including your skeletal muscles. This oxygen enables your muscles to create fuel, or energy, for your activities.

If you're performing aerobic exercise, you'll most likely feel warm. You'll notice your breathing rate and pulse are higher than at rest. Examples of aerobic activities include walking, jogging, dancing, tennis, cross-country skiing, elliptical or stair-stepping machines, swimming, and cycling. In contrast, anaerobic exercises are performed without oxygen. Examples include sprinting or weightlifting. In some instances, the two types may be combined. For example, "interval training" could include alternating jogging (aerobic) with sprints (anaerobic).

Do you need some motivation to engage in regular cardio exercise? Following are reasons to give aerobic exercise a try.[1]

- Helps you to keep off extra pounds or even lose weight by burning calories, which means less body fat
- Improves endurance: you'll be able to do more activities you enjoy without running out of steam as quickly
- Increases bone density (if you choose a weight-bearing activity)[1,2]
- Decreases the likelihood of premature death[2]
- Reduces the risk of heart disease and diabetes[3]
- Decreases the risk of colon and breast cancer[4,5]
- Improves cardiac function and increases the likelihood of surviving a heart attack[1]
- Better mental health: regular exercise promotes the release of endorphins (our body's natural painkillers). This helps to improve mood. It also helps to decrease anxiety and depression as well as arthritis-related pain.
- Lowers moderately high blood pressure[6,7]
- Decreases resting heart rate[7]
- May improve balance, which reduces fall risk and makes it easier to perform everyday activities
- Improves the immune system, making you less likely to get colds and other viruses

- Increases HDL (good cholesterol)
- Decreases triglycerides (fat in the blood)
- Improves glucose tolerance and decreases insulin resistance: this is especially important for pre-diabetics and diabetics, for it helps them to better regulate the disease. It helps to decrease the risk that people without diabetes will get it.[2]
- Decreases fatigue
- Improves sleep
- Keeps muscles strong, which may help you stay active and independent

Wow! That's a lot of great reasons. Now that you know why it's a good idea to start an aerobic exercise program and say goodbye to being a couch potato, let's take a look at what you can do to prepare. Let's return for a moment to Jerry Brown, who we first met earlier in this chapter.

Jerry is serious about getting into shape. He looks down at his feet (or at least tries to, but it's hard to see past his middle section). He doesn't own sneakers, and he knows his old sandals aren't made for walking because they lack arch supports. He realizes he needs to invest in a pair of athletic shoes if he wants to make a real go of this. He also knows he should see his physician before starting an exercise program. Besides being overweight, he recognizes that he might have high blood pressure. His mother and one of his brothers have diabetes, and he worries that he might be next. He quit smoking two years ago and is concerned he may have done damage to his lungs. He pulls out his cell phone and dials his primary care doctor.

It's a good idea to consult your physician before you start an aerobic exercise program. This is especially the case if you're over 40, sedentary, overweight, have a history of cardiac problems, diabetes or stroke, and if you drink or smoke.

Next, pick an aerobic activity that you enjoy or that you think you'll be able to stick with. Get a pair of comfortable, supportive sneakers. Aim to exercise 3 to 5 times a week. If you haven't exercised regularly before, you may want to start with 5-10 minutes and gradually build up until you can tolerate 20 to 30 minutes at a moderate intensity. Be patient, for this may take several weeks or more to achieve. Start conservatively, for if you overdo it and do too much too quickly, it can lead to an injury which could slow your progress.

There are different ways to figure out your target heart rate/ level of exertion. If you already wear a heart rate tracking device (like a Fitbit), then you may choose to figure out your target heart rate based on the heart rate reserve formula. Training range is the upper and lower threshold expressed as a percent. Think of it as how hard you want to train, with a higher percent being more aggressive than a lower percent. The training range for aerobic exercise is 40% to 85%. The training rate is used in conjunction with the formula for heart rate reserve to create a target heart rate during exercise.

The formula for heart rate reserve is:

220-Age=Maximal Heart Rate (Max HR)

Next, Max HR-resting HR= Heart Rate Reserve (HRR)

Then, multiply the HRR by the percent at which you want to train. Finally, add back your resting HR.

For example, assuming an age of 60, a resting heart rate of 70 beats per minute, and a 50% training rate:

220-60=160

160-70=90

90 x 50%= 90 x 0.5= 45

45+ 70= 115 beats per minute

So, in this example, a 60-year-old with a resting heart rate of 70 who wants to train at 50% would try to maintain a heart rate of 115 beats per minute while performing aerobic exercise.

Does the above math make you queasy? Don't worry. You can also rate perceived exertion by simply assessing how you feel, which correlates with your heart rate. This method is referred to as the Borg Rating of Perceived Exertion (RPE). This helps you to determine if you're working too hard or not hard enough.

When you exercise, your breathing becomes faster and deeper. Your heart rate increases. Your muscles may begin to feel tired. These are all hints that you can use to determine your rate of perceived exertion. The Borg Rating of Perceived Exertion, designed by Gunnar Borg, is based on a general feeling of how hard you feel you are exercising. (A brief side note: "Borg" is not related to the recurring antagonists who appeared in Star Trek!). Rate your exertion on a scale of 6 to 20. The reason that the scale starts with 6 is because it is designed to correlate with your resting heart rate (which is often about 60 beats per minute). So, for example, a 6 would equate with how you feel when you are standing still (no exertion at all). Seven is extremely light, 9 is very light, 11 is light, 13 is somewhat hard, 15 is hard, 17 very hard, 19 extremely hard, and 20 maximal exertion. Level 12 to 14 is considered moderate-intensity exercise. Level 15 and above is vigorous-intensity exercise.

In general, moderate intensity would be associated with an increase in breathing rate and a light sweat after 10 minutes of exercise. If you are performing a vigorous-intensity activity, your breathing becomes deep and rapid, you start sweating after a couple of minutes of exercise, and you can't speak more than a couple of words without pausing to take a breath.

If you multiply your RPE by 10, you get an estimate of your heart rate during activity. For example, if you feel your exertion is somewhat hard and rate it 13, then:

13 x 10 = 130= estimated heart rate

This rating scale is particularly helpful for people whose heart rate is affected by medications. For example, beta blockers slow down a person's heart rate. Therefore, setting a target heart rate based on pulse alone may not be a good option. The RPE would be a more accurate assessment of how hard a person is working.

Jerry Brown bends over and ties his new sneakers. His doctor gives him the green light to start exercising. He decides to start with walking in his neighborhood. It is spring, and the weather is perfect for outdoor activities.

Are you ready to try giving aerobic exercise a try? Start off by warming up at a light exertional level. This means start slowly to let your heart and muscles accommodate to the workload. Then increase your exercise intensity to the desired level. Finish your aerobic workout with a "cool-down" consisting of 3 to 5 minutes of light exercise. This helps avoid pooling of blood in your legs, which can occur if you stop suddenly during or after vigorous exercise. Skipping a proper cool-down can lead to dizziness.

You may also choose to do some light stretching after aerobic exercise. Please refer to Chapter 13 "Staying Flexible: Stretching Muscles Safely" for details about proper stretching.

The Surgeon General and the American College of Sports Medicine (ACSM) both offer suggestions regarding physical activity. The Surgeon General recommends a regular, preferably daily regimen of at least 30-45 minutes of brisk walking, bicycling, or even working around the house or yard. Activity can be obtained in longer sessions of moderately intense activities (such as walking) or in shorter sessions of more vigorous activities (such as fast walking or stair climbing).

The ACSM recommends engaging in moderate-intensity cardiorespiratory exercise for 30 or more minutes on 5 or more days per week for a total of 150 or more minutes per week. Alternatively, you can choose vigorous-intensity cardiorespiratory exercise training for 20 or more minutes on 3 or more days per week, for a total of 75 or more minutes per week.

If you're sedentary, it's okay to start off with 5 minutes of exercise and gradually build up as tolerated. Even increasing your activity level in general by walking around the house and garden more, climbing the stairs more, and standing up and down from sitting is better than not exercising at all. Getting started is the hardest part.

Write down a plan for the week to get motivated and stay on track. Each day record the type of activity and how many minutes you perform it. Try to be realistic and set achievable goals. As you adjust to the exercise program, change your goals accordingly.

If you are hesitant or unsure, start slowly. You can do something as simple as walking for five minutes in the morning and five minutes in the afternoon or evening. As you gain confidence, there are many different aerobic activities to choose from, from gym classes to bicycling, jogging, tennis, or dancing. If you suffer from arthritis, you may opt to try swimming or other activities in a pool.

Below is a list of aerobic activities with the approximate number of calories burned per hour for a 150-154-pound individual who is 5'10" tall. Right now, you may be thinking how many people who are 5'10" tall weigh only 150 pounds? This is the height and weight chosen by the United States Department of Agriculture. Just keep in mind that people who weigh more will burn more calories and those who weigh less will burn fewer calories.

The activities listed below show the number of calories burned with various activities, as determined by the United States Department of Agriculture (www.choosemyplate.gov).

- Aerobics class: 480
- Basketball (vigorous): 440
- Bicycling (outdoor less than 10 mph): 290
- Bicycling (outdoor greater than 10 mph): 590
- Bicycling (stationary): 480-540
- Cross-country skiing: 530-630
- Dancing: 330
- Gardening: 330

- Golfing (Walking and carrying golf clubs): 330
- Hiking: 370
- Jogging/Running 5 mph: 590
- Jumping rope: 650-800
- Skating: 470-550
- Swimming (slow freestyle laps): 510
- Tennis: 470-550
- Volleyball: 200-240
- Yard work (heavy): 440
- Walking (3.5 mph): 280
- Walking (4.5 mph): 460
- Weight training: 220

As you try some of the activities above, get fit and have fun. It's all part of the path toward healthy aging.

Chapter 3

Tips for Lowering Your Blood Pressure

Jackson Williamson sits down and takes a deep breath. Lately, he's been under a lot of stress at home and work. When he went for a routine physical last week, his physician pointed out his blood pressure is high. His doctor told him to check his blood pressure several times each day. He is supposed to return in two weeks to discuss the readings and see if he needs blood pressure medication. He wants to avoid having to take a pill. He hopes he can lower it with changes to his diet, exercising more, and managing his stress level better.

New Guidelines for High Blood Pressure

You may have high blood pressure and not even realize it. In 2017, the American College of Cardiology and the American Heart Association lowered the threshold for diagnosis of hypertension (high blood pressure). Previously, a person was diagnosed with hypertension for blood pressure 150/80 mm of mercury (mm Hg) or greater (age 65 and older) and 140/90 (under the age of 65). The new guideline to be diagnosed with hypertension is 130/80 millimeters of mercury (mm Hg) for all adults.

What is Blood Pressure and How is it Measured?

Blood pressure is measured with a sphygmomanometer (inflatable cuff with a gauge) and stethoscope. First, the cuff is wrapped around the upper arm and is pumped up until it's inflated. A stethoscope is placed near the front of the elbow and is used to listen to when one's heartbeat can first be heard (the systolic blood pressure) and when the sound goes away or greatly diminishes (the diastolic blood pressure). If a person's blood pressure is 120/80 mm Hg, this means the systolic pressure is 120 mm Hg and the diastolic pressure is 80 mm Hg.

When your heart beats, it squeezes and pushes blood along through your arteries. The pressure (force) exerted by the blood on your artery walls is your systolic blood pressure. Normal systolic pressure is less than 120 mm Hg. According to the American Heart Association, a systolic (upper number) of:

- 120-129 mm Hg = elevated.
- 130-139 mm Hg = stage 1 hypertension (high blood pressure)
- 140 mm Hg or more = stage 2 hypertension (high blood pressure)
- 180 mm Hg or more = a hypertensive crisis (get emergency assistance)

When your heart relaxes, it fills with blood. The force exerted on the artery walls while the heart is resting is your diastolic blood pressure. Normal diastolic blood pressure is less than 80 mm Hg. According to the American Heart Association, diastolic blood pressure of:

- 80-89 mm Hg = stage 1 hypertension (high blood pressure)
- 90 mm Hg or more = stage 2 hypertension (high blood pressure)
- 120 mm Hg or more = a hypertensive crisis (get emergency assistance)

The American Heart Association has combined the above systolic and diastolic readings such that:

Normal: Less than 120/80 mm Hg
Elevated: Systolic between 120-129 *and* diastolic less than 80
Stage 1: Systolic between 130-139 *or* diastolic between 80-89
Stage 2: Systolic at least 140 *or* diastolic at least 90 mm Hg

Hypertensive crisis: Systolic over 180 and/or diastolic over 120 (may require prompt changes to medications or immediate hospitalization depending on patient condition)

Your physician will take your blood pressure as part of your annual physical exam. If it's high, you may need to have it monitored more frequently. Some people choose to buy a home blood pressure machine. We'll discuss choosing a home machine and how to accurately measure blood pressure a little later in this chapter.

Sometimes, a person's blood pressure goes up only when a medical professional takes a reading. This is called "white-coat hypertension." If you are susceptible to this problem, it's helpful to get a home blood pressure unit so that you can compare your readings with the ones taken by your health care professional.

If you have an elevated reading, your doctor may suggest lifestyle changes. If you have State I hypertension with a history of diabetes, chronic kidney disease, stroke, heart attack, or other cardiovascular problems (or if you're at high risk for having one of these conditions), your physician may prescribe medication. Patients with Stage II hypertension may also be prescribed medications. Sometimes, two or more types may be required to control blood pressure. Healthy aging requires being aware of your blood pressure and addressing it as needed. Even if a person's blood pressure is high, it's common not to have any symptoms. For this reason, hypertension is often referred to as "the silent killer." The first symptom of high blood pressure can be a stroke or heart attack. In the next section, we'll take a look at some things you can do to lower your blood pressure or keep it in the normal range as you get older.

Tips for Lowering Your Blood Pressure

The first step to taking charge of your blood pressure is to learn how to measure it. Invest in a home blood pressure monitor, which ranges in price from about $40 to $100. Sometimes, insurance may cover part or all the cost. Purchase a unit with a bright, easy-to-see digital readout. Some monitors can send your readings wirelessly to your smartphone via an app. Others can plug into your smartphone to transfer data.

It's best to get one with an automatic inflating cuff. If you purchase a home unit, keep in mind that cuffs that go around the upper arm tend to be more accurate than those that go around the forearm/wrist or a finger. Make sure the cuff is the right size for your arm. If the cuff is too small, it may result in a reading that is higher than your actual blood pressure.

Closely follow the directions on the unit. To ensure accuracy, it's a good idea to bring it to your health care provider's office and compare readings between your blood pressure monitor and your physician's.

Avoid smoking or drinking caffeine for 30 minutes prior to taking your blood pressure. Also, sit and rest quietly for five minutes before taking it. For an accurate reading, sit with your back supported and your feet flat on the floor (don't cross your legs). Place the cuff on bare skin. Make sure your arm is supported and elevated to the level of your heart. For example, you can rest it on a table but place a pillow under your arm if you need to make it higher. If you have questions, your medical provider can demonstrate proper positioning.

Depending on your needs and your doctor's advice, measure your blood pressure a few times per week. Keep a journal, including the time and blood pressure reading. If you get an abnormal reading, rest a minute and repeat taking the blood pressure.

People can often lower their blood pressure by making lifestyle changes:

- Eat a well-balanced, low-salt diet, such as the DASH diet. The daily recommended value for sodium is less than 2,300 mg per day (some recommend an even lower threshold of 1,500 mg per day). Beware of processed foods and restaurant foods, which can be high in sodium. Choose deli meats and soups that are clearly marketed as low in sodium. Decreasing salt intake may lower your systolic blood pressure by 5-11 points.

- Increase your potassium intake. According to the National Institute of Health, females should strive for 2,600 mg per day and males 3,400 mg daily. This may decrease your systolic pressure by 4-5 points.

- Exercise regularly. Include both aerobic exercise (90 to 150 minutes per week) and resistance training. Consistent exercise may lead to a 5-point drop in systolic pressure. [1]

- Maintain a healthy weight. For every two pounds you lose, you may see a 1-point drop in systolic blood pressure.[1]

- Manage stress. Please refer to Part V: Wellness for further details.

- Limit alcohol to one drink a day for women and two for men. This can decrease your systolic blood pressure by up to 4 points.

- Quit smoking.

Following these steps can help you to keep your blood pressure in the normal range as you get older. If you have elevated blood pressure, following these strategies may help you to stay off medications. If you require medications, you may be able to take lower doses or a milder medication.

Chapter 4

What You Should Know about Strokes

Glenda gazes into the mirror as she brushes her teeth. Suddenly, one side of her face begins drooping. Toothpaste leaks out of the corner of her mouth. She wants to wipe it away with her right hand, but when she tries, she can't reach her mouth. Instead, her arm drops weakly down to her side. She staggers to her bedroom and collapses into a chair. "Help!" she calls out. Her sister rushes in to see what's wrong. Glenda tries to explain but finds it difficult to get the words out.

A stroke occurs when blood flow to a part of the brain is cut off. A stroke can also be referred to as "brain attack" or cerebrovascular accident (CVA). It can be caused by the rupture of an artery to the brain (hemorrhagic stroke) or a blockage of blood flow in the brain (ischemic stroke). If brain cells do not receive oxygen, they begin to die. When these cells die during a stroke, the tasks controlled by that region of the brain are lost. For example, depending on what area of the brain is affected, a person may lose their ability to speak, understand language, use their muscles, or even their sense of balance. If the area impacted is small, the stroke may result in minor deficits. Likewise, a large stroke can cause paralysis or loss of speech.

According to the National Stroke Association, stroke is the leading cause of adult disability in the United States. Moreover, two-thirds of all strokes cause some sort of disability. Their website, www.stroke.org, provides the following statistics regarding strokes:

- Nearly 800,000 people experience a new or recurrent stroke each year.
- A stroke occurs every 40 seconds.
- Stroke is the fifth leading cause of death in the U.S.
- Someone dies from a stroke every 4 minutes.

Risk Factors for Stroke

A risk factor is something that increases your chances of having a condition, such as a stroke. Some risk factors can be controlled, while others cannot. If you are aware of your risk factors for having a stroke, it can better prepare you for action in case you recognize the signs in yourself or a loved one. Knowledge of risk factors can also assist you in figuring out how to lower your risk.

The most important risk factor for stroke is hypertension, also known as high blood pressure. Normal blood pressure is 120/80 mmHg. Please refer to Chapter 3 for detailed information about hypertension. Other risk factors that can be controlled include high cholesterol, diabetes, and smoking.

A buildup of plaque in your carotid arteries (located in your neck) can lead to stroke. Atrial fibrillation, which is an abnormal heart rhythm marked by a rapid, irregular heart rate which arises from the atrial myocardium (upper chambers of the heart muscle), increases stroke risk fivefold. Blood clotting disorders and sleep apnea are additional risk factors. Other factors which you can control include excessive drinking and use of drugs, such as heroin and cocaine. Obesity and physical inactivity can also play a role. In addition, use of birth control in women may increase risk.

A transient ischemic attack (TIA) is similar to a stroke, but the effects don't last more than 24 hours. For this reason, they are sometimes referred to as "ministrokes." Since the blockage of blood flow to the brain is temporary, there's no permanent damage. However, it can be a warning sign of a future stroke. According to the National Stroke Association, approximately one-third of people who experience a TIA but don't seek treatment will suffer a more severe stroke within one year. Bottom line: if you suspect you are having a TIA, get appropriate treatment immediately to reduce future stroke risk.

Some risk factors can't be controlled. Examples include gender (women have a higher risk than men, partly because they live longer) and age (your risk increases as you get older). If you've suffered a stroke in the past, this increases your odds of having another one.

I recently responded with my volunteer rescue squad to a first aid call for an elderly male suffering a possible cerebrovascular accident. When we arrived, our patient (I'll call him Harold) explained to us that he felt fine when he woke up that morning. He showered, brushed his teeth, and got dressed. As he walked down the stairs, he noticed that his right leg felt weak. When he reached up into a kitchen cabinet to grab his coffee mug, he discovered his arm also felt weak. While chatting with his wife, he realized that he knew what he wanted to say but felt like his speech was slurred. "I felt like I was drunk," he said.

Harold's wife suggested that she call 911, but her husband refused. "Honestly, I thought the weakness would go away on its own," he explained to us.

They went to a dinner party and one of Harold's friends noticed that he seemed "off" somehow. The friend suggested he call his doctor, but Harold declined. "I'm sure I'll be fine."

It wasn't until ten o'clock that night that Harold finally relented to his family's desire for him to go to the emergency room. By that time, he'd delayed receiving care for 14 hours. Is this a big deal? YES. I'll explain why below.

As a volunteer emergency medical technician (EMT), I've responded to hundreds of calls for people suffering from cerebrovascular accidents. As a physical therapist working in the hospital and outpatient settings, I've treated countless victims of stroke. Many times, I think to myself, *if only someone had called 911 sooner.* Healthy aging includes being aware of the warning signs of stroke and knowing what to do if you or a loved one experience them. Every minute following a stroke is of vital importance. Do not waste one precious moment. Get help immediately.

Warning signs of a stroke can come on gradually or start suddenly. Signs of a stroke may include:

- Weakness and/or numbness of your face, arm, or leg. The weakness is often on only one side of the body.
- Difficulty speaking (confusion, trouble speaking, or difficulty understanding speech)
- Feeling confused or having trouble understanding others
- Trouble seeing with one or both eyes
- Headache, which may come on suddenly and be severe
- Difficulty walking, possibly with decreased balance and coordination
- Dizziness

If you think someone may be having a stroke, The American Stroke Association (www.stroke association.org) advocates using the acronym "FAST."

FACE DROOPING: Does one side of the person's face droop? Is one side of the face numb? Ask the person to smile. Is the smile asymmetrical or lopsided?

ARM WEAKNESS: Ask the person to raise both arms overhead. Does one arm go up higher than the other? Does the person have trouble keeping one of the arms up? Is one arm weak or numb?

SPEECH DIFFICULTY: Ask the person to repeat a short, simple phrase. Does he or she slur their words? Are you able to understand them? Does he have difficulty repeating a simple phrase back to you?

TIME TO CALL 911: If the answer to any of the above questions is YES, call 911 IMMEDIATELY! If you aren't sure, call 911. Even if the symptoms go away, you should still call 911.

An updated variation of FAST is BE FAST. This adds B for Balance and E for Eyes to the acronym.

BALANCE: Look for a sudden loss of balance or coordination. This may be evident when the person stands up and tries to walk.

EYES: Does the person have a sudden loss of vision, double vision, or blurred vision?

Make sure you take note of the time when the symptoms first appeared. Important medical treatment decisions may need to be based on this information. For example, tissue plasminogen activator (commonly called tPA) is a "clot-buster," meaning it's a drug used to treat strokes by dissolving blood clots. It must be administered within 3 hours (and sometimes up to 4.5 hours) of when a person first shows signs of having a stroke. To receive this drug, you must first undergo testing to make sure your stroke is due to a clot rather than a hemorrhage (brain bleed). The sooner you seek help when you show signs of a stroke, the better.

How to Decrease Your Risk of Stroke

According to the National Stroke Association, up to 80 percent of strokes can be prevented. How can you go about reducing your risk of stroke? Do any of the risk factors outlined in the previous chapter apply to you? Knowing your own risk factors is an important part of staying healthy. It allows you to take steps to decrease your stroke risk.

For starters, see your physician for a wellness check. Hypertension is the number one risk factor for stroke. Find out if your blood pressure is normal. If it's high, your doctor will address it. If you are prescribed medication, make sure to take it as directed.

According to the American Stroke Association, diabetes doubles your risk of stroke. If you have diabetes or blood sugar issues, make sure they're adequately controlled. Since high cholesterol increases the risk for plaque and clots, it raises your stroke risk. If your cholesterol levels are elevated, make sure to follow your physician's advice. Sleep apnea also increases stroke risk, so those who suffer from it should also be under the care of a physician.

Smoking damages blood vessels, which can increase your risk of stroke. If you smoke, ask your physician to help you quit. If you live with smokers, encourage them to stop smoking.

Likewise, if you drink excessively, cut back. According to the American Stroke Association, drinking more than one drink per day in women and two drinks a day in men increases blood pressure, which in turn increases stroke risk. Avoid the use of illegal drugs, as they also increase stroke risk.

Eat a healthy, well-balanced diet. Exercise regularly and keep your weight in an acceptable range for your height. In addition, seek medical assistance if you find you have difficulty managing your stress level. These topics will be discussed in more detail in upcoming chapters.

Chapter 5

Heart Health and Chest Pain

*B*ob *Smith lets out a loud belch. It tastes reminiscent of the onions on the bacon cheeseburger he ate earlier that evening. He knows he ate too much. Besides the burger, he'd chowed down a large order of fries, a bunch of chicken nuggets, and a milkshake. Now, he has a serious case of indigestion. Or at least that's what he thinks it is. He began burping an hour ago, and now he's beginning to wonder if it could be something more sinister than acid reflux. At first, he thinks the pain is in his stomach, but now it's moving up to his chest. Beads of cold sweat break out across his forehead. He begins feeling nauseated and quickly pops another antacid pill into his mouth. He contemplates taking aspirin as well. He stares at the phone, uncertain whether to call 911. Could he be having a heart attack? He doesn't want to go to the hospital if it's just a case of indigestion.*

In my years as a volunteer emergency medical technician, I've witnessed numerous people wrestle with the question posed above. It can be very confusing to determine the difference between indigestion and a myocardial infarction, commonly referred to as an MI or heart attack. Sometimes, people may deny they could be having a heart attack.

Here are a few sobering statistics. About every 40 seconds, someone in the United States has a myocardial infarction.[1] In other words, every year, about 790,000 Americans suffer an MI.[1]

The heart, which is a muscular organ, requires oxygen. If a person has a heart attack, the blood flow to the heart is extremely decreased or cut off. How does this happen?

The arteries that supply blood to your heart are called coronary arteries. These can become narrowed or completely blocked from atherosclerosis, which is plaque made up of fat, cholesterol, and other substances that gradually build up within blood vessels. If plaque breaks away from the artery wall, a blood clot forms around it. If the clot blocks blood flow to the heart muscle, it deprives it of oxygen and nutrients. This is called ischemia. Ischemia can cause damage or death to the heart muscle. When this occurs, it is called a myocardial infarction or heart attack. Another cause of MI can be a severe spasm of a coronary artery, which stops blood flow to the heart muscle.

Besides myocardial infarction, heart attacks can also be called by other names such as acute coronary syndrome, STEMI, NSTEMI, coronary thrombosis, and coronary occlusion. Sometimes, they are named by the type of MI. For example, an ST-elevation myocardial infarction (STEMI) is a type of heart attack in which a coronary artery is completely blocked. Similarly, a non-ST-elevated myocardial infarction (NSTEMI) occurs when an artery is partially blocked, leading to greatly reduced blood flow.

One out of five heart attacks are silent, meaning the person is not aware he or she had a myocardial infarction.[1] This is more common in people who have diabetes. Oftentimes, there are indicators that a heart attack is occurring. Bear in mind that symptoms can vary from person to person. The more symptoms you have, the more likely you're having an MI. By knowing the signs and symptoms, you can seek help right away.

You can also have chest pains without having a heart attack. Angina pectoris is a common type of recurring chest discomfort that usually lasts only a few minutes. It commonly occurs during activity or emotional stress when your heart muscle needs more oxygen but isn't getting a sufficient amount. Angina doesn't permanently damage the heart muscle.

Warning Signs of a Heart Attack

- Chest pain: Pain may be mild to severe in nature. It can come on suddenly or gradually.
- Chest pressure or discomfort: People may feel like there is an "elephant on their chest." They may complain of a sensation of fullness, squeezing, or pressure, typically in the left or central chest.
- Complaint of "heartburn"
- Pain in other parts of the body, such as the neck, jaw, back, upper stomach, shoulders, and arms (left more so than right, but it can even be either or both arms)
- Shortness of breath, possibly with coughing or wheezing
- Breaking out into a cold sweat
- Anxiety
- Fatigue
- Nausea/vomiting
- Lightheadedness or dizziness

Like men, the most common heart attack symptom in women is chest pain or discomfort. However, women may be more likely to experience other common symptoms, including jaw/back pain, nausea and/or vomiting, and difficulty breathing or shortness of breath.

Now you know how to identify the warning signs of a heart attack in yourself or others. In the next section, we'll review the risk factors for myocardial infarctions.

Know the Risk Factors for a Heart Attack

Let's check back in with Bob Smith, who we first met earlier in the chapter.

Bob says a prayer of thanks each morning that he survived the heart attack that threatened to end his life just a few short weeks after celebrating his fiftieth birthday. His father died from a massive heart attack at the age of forty-six. Given his family history, Bob realizes he should have gone to a cardiologist for a check-up years ago. Being an overweight smoker has further increased his odds of having "the big one." He vows to make a change in his lifestyle.

Risk factors increase your likelihood of developing coronary heart disease and heart attacks. Some risks you can't change, like age (45 and older for males and 55 and older for females) and gender (being male). Males are more likely to suffer a heart attack, but women who are older than 65 are more likely to die from one. Another risk factor that you can't control is family history. You are more likely to have a heart attack if you have a sibling, parents, or grandparents who had an early heart attack (age 65 or younger for females and 55 or younger for males). Race is also a risk factor. African Americans have a higher risk, possibly related to hypertension.

Some risk factors can be controlled. Recall that atherosclerosis is the buildup of fatty deposits within your arteries. It increases your risk of a heart attack. By working with your physician, you can strive to decrease or prevent atherosclerosis.

Other risk factors that can be modified include:

- **Smoking/tobacco use:** Do you really need another reason to quit? Smoking and prolonged exposure to secondhand smoke increase MI risk.
- **High blood pressure**. Hypertension over a period of time can damage your arteries, including those that supply your heart

with blood. This can lead to a faster build-up of plaque in the arteries.

- **High blood cholesterol or triglyceride levels:** Elevated levels of low-density lipoprotein (LDL) cholesterol (sometimes referred to as "bad" cholesterol) may lead to a narrowing of arteries. Triglycerides are a type of diet-related fat in the blood. High levels of triglycerides increase your risk of heart attack. In contrast, a high level of high-density lipoprotein (HDL) cholesterol (known as "good" cholesterol) lowers your risk.

- **Diabetes:** Your body needs glucose, a form of sugar, to function. The pancreas secretes insulin, a hormone which enables you to be able to utilize glucose. Diabetes is a condition in which the body does not produce adequate insulin or doesn't respond to insulin levels properly. This may cause your body's blood sugar levels to rise above or fall below normal. Diabetes, especially when it is not adequately controlled, increases your risk of having a heart attack.

- **Lack of physical activity:** A sedentary lifestyle may lead to high blood cholesterol levels, decreased cardiovascular fitness, and obesity. Aerobic exercise improves cardiovascular fitness and helps to lower blood pressure, which decreases overall risk of heart attack. Exercise is also beneficial in lowering high blood pressure.

- **Obesity:** Being overweight may lead to high blood cholesterol levels, high triglyceride levels, diabetes, and hypertension. Losing weight can lower your risk.

- **Drug abuse:** Stimulant drugs, like amphetamines or cocaine, can cause a spasm of your coronary arteries that may trigger a myocardial infarction.

- **Stress:** Your body's reaction to stress may increase your risk of a heart attack.

To decrease your risk, first figure out your risk factors for a heart attack and modify the ones you can. Prevention is key. For starters, if you smoke, quit. If you have high blood pressure, high cholesterol, or diabetes, work with your physician to manage them. Eating healthy, striving to be active and fit, and maintaining a healthy weight are important steps to decreasing your risk.

What to Do if you Suddenly Experience Chest Pain

The previous two sections describe what causes heart attacks and risk factors that make you more susceptible. Now it's time to learn what to do if you suddenly experience chest pains.

- **Call 911.** Don't try to wait it out to see if the pain goes away. Don't assume it's just an upset stomach. Let trained medical personnel transport you to the hospital. Drive yourself only as a last resort since your condition could worsen, placing you at risk of injuring yourself or others.
- **Chew a regular-strength (325 mg) aspirin.** A baby aspirin is 81mg, so you would have to chew four baby aspirin to equal one adult dose. Aspirin reduces blood clotting. This may allow some blood to flow around the area of the coronary artery that is narrowed by a clot or plaque (i.e., the region causing the myocardial infarction). Don't take aspirin if you're already on a blood thinner, such as Coumadin (generic name warfarin). Also, don't take aspirin if you're allergic to it or if your physician has previously advised against it.
- **If your doctor has prescribed nitroglycerin for you, now is the time to take it.** Nitroglycerin widens your blood vessels, which allows increased blood flow. Make sure not to take someone else's nitroglycerin.

What if it's a loved one or friend complaining of chest pain? You can help by following the steps above. If you're trained in performing cardiopulmonary resuscitation (CPR) and the person falls unconscious and has no pulse, begin CPR with chest compressions. If you're not certified in CPR and don't know what to do, the 911 dispatcher can talk you through the steps.

Don't worry about giving mouth-to-mouth breathing. Many people do not want to perform rescue breathing on a stranger due to the risk of acquiring an infection. It's recommended that bystanders who are not trained in CPR perform chest compressions only (without rescue breathing) at a rate of 100 to 120 compressions per minute.

Nowadays, automated external defibrillators (AEDs) can often be found in many public places, such as government buildings, stadiums, schools, as well as churches. If you have access to an automated external defibrillator (AED), follow the device's instructions. You do not need to be certified to use a defibrillator. The AED should provide voice prompts to guide you through the steps. There are few things more rewarding than playing a role in resuscitating a person in cardiac arrest and giving them a new lease on life.

Learn CPR and the Heimlich Maneuver

This topic is near and dear to my heart. As a volunteer EMT, I've responded to hundreds of calls for people who were choking or in cardiac arrest. Thanks to first responders and bystanders who took the time to learn how to help choking victims and those who suffer sudden cardiac death, many of these people are alive today.

You may be wondering, *how is learning cardiopulmonary resuscitation (CPR) going to make me healthier?* Technically, I suppose it isn't. BUT, if enough people learn CPR and the Heimlich maneuver, it just may help you or a loved one, should you ever need it. CPR isn't just for victims of

33

cardiac emergencies. People who choke can become unresponsive and may need CPR as well.

Over 4,000 people die from choking each year in the United States. [2] In 2017, the number climbed to 5,216.[3] According to the National Safety Council, choking was the fourth leading cause of unintentional death in the United Stated in 2017.[4]

Sometimes, people who are choking feel embarrassed and don't want to draw attention to themselves. I've responded to numerous first aid calls at restaurants in which choking victims became unresponsive as they rushed to the bathroom to cough out the object in private. To make matters worse, if a person is found unconscious in a restroom, people may assume the victim suffered a heart attack. This could delay life-saving chest thrusts.

Wearing dentures or having difficulty swallowing can increase choking risk. The universal sign for choking is putting one or both hands to the throat. Signs of choking include clutching the throat, coughing, gagging, wheezing, and passing out.

A choking victim can have a partial or complete airway obstruction. A person with a partial (mild) obstruction can cough and make sounds. Let the person cough to expel the object. If you have concerns about the person's airway or breathing, call 911.

In contrast, a person with a complete airway obstruction won't be able to cough effectively. If you find a person in distress who cannot cough, speak, or make sounds, or who cannot breathe, or is making the universal sign for choking, it's time to take quick action by performing the Heimlich maneuver. The Heimlich maneuver uses quick abdominal (belly) thrusts to act like a cough by forcing air from the lungs. This may help to expel the object from the airway.

Picture this. You're out to lunch with a group of co-workers. Your friend John pops a big wad of mozzarella cheese into his mouth. Suddenly, he gets a panicked look on his face and clutches his hands to his throat. What do you do?

Steps to Perform the Heimlich Maneuver for a Conscious Adult Choking Person

1. Confirm that the person cannot cough or speak. Tell him that you are going to help.
2. Stand behind the patient. Try to stagger your feet by placing one foot in between the victim's legs and the other foot behind you. This way, if he falls unconscious, you are in a good position to lower him to the floor. (If your feet are close together and the patient collapses to the ground, it could pull you down as well).
3. Wrap your arms around him so that your hands are in front of his belly.
4. Make a fist with one hand and place the thumb-side of the fist just above the belly button (navel) and well below the tip of the person's breastbone (sternum).
5. Grasp your fist with your other hand.
6. Give quick upward and inward thrusts into the person's belly.
7. Keep giving thrusts until the object comes out, the person can cough, speak, or breathe, or until he falls unconscious.

Note: if a person is pregnant or too large for you to wrap your arms around, then follow the steps above except wrap your arms around their chest, such that your fist is on the lower half of the victim's breastbone. Then administer chest thrusts until the person recovers or becomes unresponsive.

If a person falls unconscious or stops responding, lower him to the floor onto his back, such that he is face up. Instruct a bystander to call 911. Begin performing chest compressions until the person recovers or someone with more training, such as Emergency Medical Services (EMS), arrives and takes over.

Describing how to perform CPR is beyond the scope of this book. The American Heart Association and the American Red Cross offer courses to teach people how to perform CPR and the Heimlich maneuver. Just a few short hours of training will give you the tools to take life-saving action to help others. As a volunteer EMT, I've been blessed to assist numerous choking victims. However, the first two times that I performed the Heimlich maneuver, I wasn't with the rescue squad. The first time I performed the technique was on my own father. The next time occurred when my husband and I were celebrating the first night of our honeymoon in a restaurant. A woman at the next table began yelling for help when her husband began choking. Over the years, I can honestly say that some of the most rewarding moments in my life include the times I was able to help others.

If aiding others isn't enough to motivate you, consider this. According to the National Safety Council's *Injury Facts 2017*, your odds of choking to death are about 1 in 2,696.[2] If you are ever unfortunate enough to choke, you can do the Heimlich maneuver on yourself. Place the thumb side of your fist against your abdomen, just above your belly button. Then repeatedly thrust yourself against a hard object, such as the back of a hard chair or the edge of a table, until you expel the object from your airway.

Chapter 6

Keep the Pounds Off: Avoiding Weight Gain

Olga sucks in her stomach as she tries buttoning her shorts. It's no use. She pulls them off and looks in her drawers for a pair of shorts with an elastic waistband. Extra pounds have slowly been creeping onto her waist and remaining there with annoying tenacity. Gaining one pound a year doesn't seem bad, but now twenty years later, she thinks she looks six months pregnant. She knows it must be bad for her heart to carry so much extra weight in her mid-section.

Do you think that gaining weight is an unavoidable part of aging? That a bulging waistline is inevitable? Well, it doesn't have to be.

You may wonder why it becomes easier to pack on pounds as you creep into middle age and beyond. Age-related weight gain occurs when the amount of muscle decreases while the proportion of fat increases. Dropping hormone levels may contribute to loss of muscle. This change in body composition slows down metabolism, which in turn makes it easier to gain weight. When muscles work, they burn calories. So, less muscle tissue equals less calories burned.

In addition, some people become less active as they age. If a person eats the same amount as he did when he was younger, but exercises less, he'll gain weight. The pounds may slowly sneak on. Even if it's only one pound a year starting at age fifty, that's ten pounds in a decade. Before you know it, you could find yourself like Olga in the vignette above, sporting a twenty-pound spare tire.

We're bombarded with subtle and not-so-subtle cues to eat all day long, from radio and TV commercials, while shopping, and when seeing others consume food. Sometimes, it may seem impossible to resist.

Perhaps you may find yourself indulging before you even realize it. Before grabbing an unhealthy snack or reaching for a second helping, pause and ask yourself, "Am I really hungry?" Eating can be due to habit or the power of suggestion, rather than true need. Mindless eating while watching a movie or sporting event can lead to unwanted weight gain.

Being overweight can increase the risk of getting diabetes, cancer, and sleep apnea. Obesity increases the odds of getting high blood pressure and other heart conditions. A large waistline increases the risk of premature death.[1] One study which compared people with the same body mass index found that the risk of premature death increased in a linear fashion as waist circumference increased. The risk of premature death was almost double for subjects with a larger waist (more than 47.2 inches for men and more than 39.4 inches for women) compared to subjects with a smaller waist (less than 31.5 inches for men and less than 25.6 inches for women).

Certain habits can lead to "tight pants." Avoiding exercise and drinking sweetened drinks can contribute to weight gain. Replace sodas and sweetened beverages with water. Try drinking coffee or tea without adding cream or sugar.

Likewise, choosing simple carbs over whole grain foods can lead to extra pounds. Start your day by eating a healthy breakfast. Whole grain foods and protein tend to be more satisfying and will curb your hunger longer than simple carbs and white grains like white rice and white bread. Fruits and veggies make a healthier snack than chips, cookies, and soda.

If you're having cereal for breakfast, choose one that's high in fiber and add low-fat dairy or almond milk. Toss in a handful of berries or other fruit on the side. If you prefer toast, choose whole-grain bread, and consider topping it with vegetables, like freshly sliced tomatoes or avocados. Eggs, a good source of protein, can also be part of a healthy breakfast. A smoothie, rich with fruits and veggies, can also be on your menu.

When building a lunchtime sandwich, choose whole grain bread and make sure to add lettuce and tomatoes. Consider mustard, light mayonnaise, or even a sprinkle of olive oil instead of more fattening alternatives, like butter or regular mayo. Personally, I love spreading a tablespoon of organic extra virgin olive oil on a slice of 12-grain toast. If you want cheese, choose one that's low in fat. You can even skip the bread and use a slice of romaine lettuce as an alternative. When eating salad for lunch, avoid croutons and sprinkle on a vinaigrette instead of creamy dressings.

How about snack time? It's important to control portion size. Put the suggested serving size in a bowl or plate rather than eating straight from the bag. When possible, choose fruits, vegetables, or a handful of nuts. Popcorn dusted with a sprinkle of olive oil is tasty and a good source of fiber.

There are also strategies you can use at dinnertime to avoid unnecessary calories. For example, try cooking with a healthy oil rather than butter. Sprinkling vinegar and olive oil on your salad may be a healthier option than commercial dressings. Avoid trans-fat.

The more vegetables you eat, the better. Try to choose ones with different colors. Flavor veggies with fresh lemon rather than butter, oil, or cheese. Potato chips and French fries don't count as vegetables!

Choose fish and poultry over red meat, bacon, and processed meats. A serving of meat or fish should be approximately the size of a deck of cards (3 to 4 ounces).

When dining out, avoid "super-sizing" it. Choose a healthy appetizer over a fattening one. If you're craving a glass of alcohol, there's less calories in wine or a light beer than a sugary, fruit-based cocktail. For pasta lovers, incorporate a healthy vegetable sauce rather than a calorie-laden cream sauce.

One way to combat weight gain is to perform resistance training 2-3 times per week. (More to come on this in upcoming chapters). Building muscle mass helps you to both burn calories and prevent muscle tissue from being replaced with fat. A small investment in your time for just a few days each week can result in better health now and in years to come.

Another means of fighting weight gain is to avoid the following unhealthy habits.

- Not making time for physical activity
- Reaching for second helpings before you have a chance for your meal to settle
- Finishing your children's meals
- Mindless snacking while watching television or surfing the internet
- Skipping breakfast

Cardiovascular exercise is another method of preventing a burgeoning waistline. Fill up on low-calorie foods, such as fruits and vegetables. Healthy proteins, like nuts, poultry, and low-fat dairy can also help control hunger. Keep a journal of what you eat. Sometimes, just knowing you have to write down the unhealthy snack you are about to eat is enough to help you to curb the impulse.

Remember, weight gain is not an inevitable part of aging. Now, let's take a closer look at two popular, healthy diets.

"DASH" to a Healthy Diet

DASH stands for "dietary approaches to stop hypertension." The DASH diet is endorsed by the National Heart, Lung, and Blood Institute (NHLBI) as a means to lower blood pressure (https://www.nhlbi.nih.gov/). However, it's also helpful to improve heart health, decrease stroke risk, manage diabetes, and even lose weight. In 2018, US News & World Report ranked DASH tied for first place "Best Diet Overall," "Best Diet for Healthy Eating," and "Best Heart-Healthy Diet."

The DASH diet emphasizes eating fruits and vegetables, grains, low-fat dairy, legumes, and nuts. It also includes poultry, fish, and lean meat as well as healthy oils and fats (polyunsaturated and monounsaturated). This healthy diet includes foods that are high in potassium, calcium, fiber, and magnesium while at the same time limiting sodium to 2,300 mg a day (some even suggest 1,500 mg daily). This, in turn, helps to lower blood pressure.

DASH discourages people from eating red meats, foods that are high in saturated fats, and full-fat dairy foods. It suggests cutting back on sweets, added sugars, and sweetened beverages.

Scientists supported by the NHLBI emphasize a DASH diet (based on consuming 2,100 calories per day) to include:

Total Fat= 27% of calories
Saturated fat=6% of calories
Protein=18% of calories
Carbohydrate=55% of calories

Potassium helps conduct nerve impulses and muscle contractions, regulates the flow of fluids and nutrients into and out of body cells, and helps keep your blood pressure in check by countering the effects of sodium. Most Americans fall short of the recommended daily value of 2,600 mg (females) and 3,400 mg (males). What are some potassium-rich foods? Fruits like apricots, bananas, melon, mango, oranges, and pears as well as vegetables like potatoes, tomatoes, spinach, kale, romaine lettuce, mushrooms, cucumbers, broccoli, and raw carrots. Nuts, seeds, milk, and yogurt are also great sources of potassium.

"Your Guide to Lowering Your Blood Pressure with Dash" is a 64-page booklet by the NHLBI available for free online.[3] It includes detailed information about the diet, research, sample daily meal plans, and recipes. Invest a few moments of your time to check out this worthwhile resource.

The Mediterranean Diet for Heart Health

Another tried-and-true diet option is the Mediterranean Diet. It's not a diet in the sense of a method of eating to lose weight. Rather, it's a lifestyle that incorporates healthy eating, exercise/activity, and socializing with family and friends. It gets its name from being based on Mediterranean-style cooking found in countries such as Greece, Spain, and southern Italy.

The Mediterranean Diet is associated with decreased risk of heart disease as well as cardiovascular mortality. The PREDIMED Study followed 7,447 individuals on the Mediterranean Diet. *The New England Journal of Medicine* retracted the original 2013 study due to finding an error in the process by which they randomized participants to the groups.[2] When the researchers re-analyzed the data and re-published the study in 2018, they still found a substantial decrease in cardiovascular disease, a reduction of low-density lipoproteins (LDL) cholesterol, and a decreased risk of type II diabetes.

Do you need any more reasons to give the Mediterranean Diet a try? Research has also indicated that it's associated with a decreased risk of cancer, Parkinson's disease, and Alzheimer's disease. This style of eating has also been found to decrease inflammation in the body. The cornerstone of the Mediterranean Diet is plant-based foods.

- Fruits and vegetables, which are rich in antioxidants, play an important role and should be included with each meal. Strive for seven to ten servings per day.
- Whole grains, including breads, cereals, and pasta, are also a key component.
- Try cooking on low to medium heat with olive oil. In addition, bread can be dipped in or drizzled with olive oil as described earlier. It's a healthier alternative than the saturated and trans fats found in butter and margarine. Olive oil contains monounsaturated fat, which may aid in LDL levels (often referred to as the "bad cholesterol"). Extra-virgin and virgin olive oils are the best choice because they provide antioxidant effects.
- Beans and legumes are emphasized as a healthy protein source.
- Snacks may include nuts, which include mostly unsaturated fats, as well as seeds. Since nuts are high in calories, they should not be eaten in large amounts. Avoid candied nuts or highly salted varieties. Choose natural peanut butter rather than the kinds that are high in hydrogenated fats.
- Fish and seafood should be eaten at least twice a week. Oily fishes, such as salmon, sardines, albacore tuna (in water), mackerel, and trout, are rich sources of omega-3 fatty acids.
- Consumption of dairy, yogurt, and cheese is encouraged, but skim and low-fat choices are strongly recommended. Three to four eggs may be eaten each week.
- Herbs and spices are an important part of the Mediterranean Diet. They are used in place of salt to flavor food.
- Eating red meat is limited to a few times per month. Avoid fatty meats such as bacon and sausage.
- Moderate consumption of wine (optional). Some research studies have linked drinking wine with a lowered risk of heart disease. This means approximately 3 ounces of wine daily for women and 5 ounces for men. If you're unsure if alcohol would be beneficial

for you, discuss it with your physician. If you have a personal or family history of alcohol abuse or liver disease, refrain from drinking. If you're not a drinker, don't start drinking just for this diet. Some research links consumption of alcohol to certain types of cancer.

- Eat sweets sparingly.
- Engage in physical activity.
- Enjoy meals with family and friends.

Following the Mediterranean Diet is a delicious eating style that can assist you on your path to healthy aging.

What are the "Clean Fifteen" and the "Dirty Dozen"?

Did you ever notice that junk food, like potato chips and other salty snacks, are cheaper than healthy alternatives, like fruits and vegetables? In an ideal world, organic fruits and vegetables would be available at affordable prices. However, this is usually not the case. Purchasing organic to avoid pesticides can put a strain on your wallet.

The Environmental Working Group (EWG) publishes a "Shoppers Guide to Pesticides in Produce" which can be downloaded from their website (https://www.ewg.org/).[4] The list, which is updated annually, contains what they have coined the "Clean Fifteen and the Dirty Dozen." The guide is based on analysis of the annual *U.S. Department of Agriculture's Pesticide Data Program (PDP) Report.*[5]

The EWG's guide is a handy reference to the fifteen least contaminated and twelve most contaminated fruits and vegetables. Numerous foods on the "Dirty Dozen" list tested positive for fifty or more chemicals. If you want to eat fruits and vegetables that are listed among the "Dirty Dozen," it may make sense to splurge and buy organic. In this way, you can reduce the amount of toxins that you consume.

Next time you're in the grocery store, take a moment to consider the EWG Guide. The EWG list varies from year to year. Check their website for the latest ranking of the safest and most contaminated fruits and vegetables. Decreasing your exposure to pesticides in food constitutes an important means by which you can strive towards healthy aging.

Part II: How to Make Your Bladder and Bowels Behave: Say Goodbye to Incontinence, Overactive Bladder, and Constipation

Chapter 7

Healthy "Waterworks": A Guide to Bladder Health
Urinary Incontinence and Urgency/Overactive Bladder, Pelvic Floor Strengthening, and Bladder Retraining

*D*o any of these vignettes sound familiar?

Brenda

Brenda dreads allergy season. Each time she coughs or sneezes, she knows drops of urine will leak into her underwear. She worries it will soak through to her pants, so she always wears a panty liner. When she goes out with friends, she tries not to laugh too hard. If she does, she knows she'll "pee her pants." She's scared to go to the gym because she's afraid she may leak. She plans to give up her aerobics class because it's too stressful worrying about wetting herself. Her urogynecologist suggested a sling procedure, but she hates the idea of surgery.

Debbie

Almost as soon as she finishes going to the bathroom, Debbie has the urge to urinate again. It's getting to the point where she's toileting every 30 to 45 minutes. She consoles herself that she can make it to the bathroom "in time" without leaking urine. However, she worries that if she pushes off the urge to go, she'll lose control and wet her pants. Lately, she feels tired and can barely stay awake. She can't get enough rest because she gets up every hour during the night to go to the bathroom.

Margaret

When Margaret pulls into her driveway, she worries about whether she'll make it inside without a major bladder accident. She knows from experience that as soon as she puts her house key in her front door lock, the urge to pee becomes so overwhelming that she can't hold the urine in. That's why she started wearing a thick incontinence pad. Sometimes, she even wears adult "incontinence underwear." She calls them adult

47

diapers. Just yesterday, she lost control and had such a bad "accident" that urine spilled down her legs. She thanked God she was home when it happened. Last week, she soaked her pants while at the grocery store. Now, she makes it a point to wear dark colored slacks and dresses when she goes out.

Judd

Judd feels like he's getting old. Ever since he broke his hip three weeks ago, he must use a walker to get around. It's slowing him down so much that he can't reach the toilet in time. His wife told him she could buy him some adult diapers, but he doesn't want any part of them. What if he starts using them and can't stop?

Urinary incontinence (UI) is the involuntary loss of urine. Some people assume that it's a natural part of aging, but it shouldn't be. According to the National Association for Continence, about 25 million Americans have daily urinary incontinence, and 33 million suffer from overactive bladder.[1] One in three women over the age of forty-five and one in two over the age of sixty-five have stress urinary incontinence (SUI).[1] Women are affected more than men and prevalence increases with age, hormonal changes, and childbirth. [2,3,4]

Over 200,000 women have surgery for SUI each year. [1] The economic cost of urinary incontinence in the United States is 69.5 billion, and people spend more than 20 billion per year on associated costs.[5] Personal cost of incontinence supplies can be as much as $900 per year![6] Although 80 percent of patients with incontinence can be cured or improved, sadly only one in twelve seek treatment.[1]

Anatomy

The bladder is an elastic, muscular sac which stores urine. Urine flows from the kidneys through the ureters into the bladder. Urine flows out of the bladder into a canal called the urethra and then out of the body. The urethral sphincter (your "internal sphincter") is used to control the flow of urine from the bladder. Similar to the bladder, the urethral sphincter is made from smooth muscle, so it is not under your conscious, volitional control. The pelvic floor muscles surround and support the urethra. For this reason, they are sometimes referred to as the external urethral sphincter.

In order to urinate, your brain must signal the muscular bladder wall to contract. This squeezes urine out of your bladder. At the same time, your brain signals the sphincters to relax. When this occurs, urine leaves the bladder through the urethra and exits the body.

The pelvic floor muscles have two types of pelvic floor muscle fibers that work together as a team. Slow-twitch fibers make up about 70% of the muscle bulk. Their job is to help you "hold on" throughout the day, like the string around a drawstring satchel. Fast-twitch fibers make up the other 30% of your pelvic floor muscle fibers. They are designed to act quickly and contract strongly. They add an extra closing force during a laugh, cough, or sneeze.

Types of UI

There are many different types of incontinence. People may have one or more types of UI at one time, which is referred to as Mixed Urinary Incontinence (MUI).

Stress Urinary Incontinence: Stress Urinary Incontinence (SUI) is the involuntary loss of urine on effort or physical exertion (e.g., lifting or sporting activities such as jumping or running) or with sneezing, coughing, or laughing. Brenda in the vignette above suffers from SUI. Urinary leakage is usually a small amount (a light pad can absorb it). It may involve sagging or weakness of the bladder neck. If there's a sudden increase in intra-abdominal pressure and a person's sphincter muscles are not strong enough to counteract it, urinary leakage results. There's a prevalence rate of 23.7% among women in the United States [2-3]

SUI is rare in males. It occurs most frequently in men who have undergone prostate surgery or who have suffered trauma. In women, risk increases with a difficult childbirth. Also, life cycle hormonal changes (especially less estrogen) can lead to SUI.

A person with SUI might not be able to stop the urine stream while toileting. He or she may not know how to contract the pelvic floor muscles. Risk factors include having an occupation that requires repeated straining/lifting or history of a difficult childbirth (tearing, episiotomy, large baby).

Urge Urinary Incontinence: Urgency Urinary Incontinence (UUI) is the complaint of involuntary loss of urine associated with urgency. Margaret in the vignette above has UUI. Urgency is a sudden, strong desire to pass urine which may be hard to control. It's caused by uncontrolled bladder muscle contractions. Leakage occurs a few seconds after the patient gets the urge to urinate and the bladder contracts. Large amounts of urine may be lost, possibly soaking the underwear or clothing. An incontinence pad may not be sufficient to absorb the urine.

Certain triggers can exacerbate UUI. One common trigger is the sound of running water. Also, when a person arrives home and anticipates going to the bathroom, she may experience urge-related urinary incontinence. It tends to occur in middle-age and older patients. It may occur in patients with urinary tract infections (UTI), diabetes, multiple sclerosis, stroke, or spinal cord injuries.

Overflow Incontinence: Patients with overflow incontinence cannot completely empty their bladders. This causes either a constantly full bladder requiring frequent urination or a constant dribbling of urine, or both. This type of incontinence is generally caused by weakened bladder muscles as a result of nerve damage from diabetes or other diseases. It can also result from the urethra being blocked due to kidney or urinary stones, tumors, an enlarged prostate in men, or a birth defect.

Functional Incontinence: Functional Incontinence refers to urine loss resulting from the inability to get to a toilet "in time," like Judd in the above vignette. The most common causes are conditions that cause immobility, such as stroke, severe arthritis, and dementia. Initially after surgery, such as a total knee or hip replacement, a person may not be able to get to the toilet as quickly as he or she could prior to the surgery. Use of bedside commodes and removal of physical obstacles leading to the bathroom may help functional incontinence.

Mixed Incontinence: Mixed incontinence involves more than one type of incontinence. The most common type is a mixture of urgency urinary incontinence and stress urinary incontinence. Overactive Bladder (OAB) is urinary urgency, usually accompanied by frequency and nocturia, with or without incontinence. Debbie in the vignette at the beginning of the chapter has OAB. It's normal to urinate 6-8 times in 24 hours, but people with OAB go more frequently. Nocturia is frequent nighttime voiding, meaning a person wakes up two or more times at night because of the need to urinate. Next, we'll take a look at how to keep your waterworks healthy.

What is "Normal" Bladder Health?

Have you ever felt like your bladder might explode if you didn't go to the bathroom? Have you wondered how much urine your bladder can hold before it has to be emptied? The bladder capacity of an adult is approximately 2 cups (16 ounces) of urine. As you get older, your bladder capacity may get smaller.

How many times does the average person go to the bathroom to urinate each day? It's normal to void about 6-8 times per day. Most people void every 3-4 hours during waking hours. Older people may need to urinate more frequently, but usually not more than every two hours.

Younger people should be able to sleep through the night without toileting because antidiuretic hormones limit the amount of urine made by the kidneys during sleep. As people get older, they make less of this hormone. This makes them produce more urine while they sleep. For this reason, it's normal for older folks to get up once from sleep to urinate. Urinating at night is affected by many factors, including how much fluid you drink before bedtime (especially if it's a caffeinated or alcoholic beverage), having poorly controlled diabetes, and taking certain medications, such as Lasix. Other factors include bladder infections or interrupted sleep. For women, pregnancy can cause increased nighttime voiding. For men, an enlarged prostate can lead to nocturia because it may press on the bladder neck, making it difficult for the urine to come out.

You shouldn't have to push or strain to empty your bladder. The urine should flow in a steady stream until the bladder is empty. It's not normal to have pain or discomfort with voiding.

Urges (signals) are felt as your bladder fills with urine, activating pressure receptors in your bladder wall. The first urge that you get to urinate is usually a "suggestion" rather than a "command." Since urges can be felt even when the bladder isn't full, you can usually safely ignore the first urge to go to the bathroom. As your bladder continues to fill with urine, the urges become more insistent. With practice, you can learn to control your urges.

Avoid going to the toilet "just in case." For example, if you know you're going out at 10AM and you plan to use the toilet before you leave, don't go to the bathroom at 9:30 AM. Instead, try pushing off voiding until closer to 10 AM. Or, if you happen to be passing by a bathroom but don't actually need to void, don't! If you go to the bathroom when you don't need to, you're training your bladder to give urges, or signals, to go to the bathroom more frequently. This can lead to increased urinary urgency and frequency. You shouldn't have to void more than every two hours. Try to urinate only when your bladder is full. In general, if you void eight or more ounces, you truly need to urinate. If you passed only 2-3 ounces of urine, you gave into a false urge. If you have urgency, try spacing your fluids throughout the day. In addition, we'll discuss bladder retraining, a behavioral technique to help with urinary urgency, frequency, and leakage in an upcoming section.

Keeping Your Waterworks Healthy

Don't rush, but rather take your time when emptying your bladder. You shouldn't have to push or strain to get urine out. Try to make sure you completely empty your bladder each time you pass urine. For women, if you feel like all the urine isn't coming out, you can perform a technique referred to as double voiding. When you finish toileting, stand up and wiggle your hips a bit. Then sit down and see if more urine comes out. Alternatively, while still seated on the toilet, lean forward as if tying your shoes, then sit upright again. Repeat three times. This places a gentle pressure on your abdomen to assist residual urine to come out.

We've talked about pushing off the urge to urinate, but don't take it to an extreme. Consistently ignoring the urge to go (waiting more than four hours between toileting during daytime hours) may not be healthy for your bladder and could increase the risk of getting a urinary tract infection.

The Effect of Diet on Bladder Health

Modifying your diet can help to control bladder problems. Certain kinds of food are irritating to the bladder, especially foods that have acidic properties. I don't recommend completely eliminating them. Instead, use moderation and experimentation to see which are the most irritating to your bladder. Let's say you discover that tomato sauce really makes you have to "go." Then a tomato-based dish may not be the best choice if you're going out to dinner and don't want to excuse yourself to run for the bathroom. Here's a list of foods that may irritate your bladder:

- Alcohol
- Artificial sweeteners
- Caffeinated beverages
- Citrus fruits and juices (e.g., orange, lemon, and grapefruit)

- Chocolate
- Coffee (both regular and decaf, but regular is more irritating)
- Cola (from caffeine and artificial sweeteners)
- Food colorings and flavorings
- Milk
- Onions
- Salsa
- Spicy foods
- Tea (regular and decaf, but regular is more irritating)
- Tomato based products
- Vinegar

In addition, smoking cigarettes is irritating to the bladder lining and can cause urgency. Also, "smoker's cough" may cause wear and tear on your pelvic floor muscles, which can contribute to stress urinary incontinence.

What is the best choice of beverage? Plain water! In addition, grape juice and apple juice are not irritating to the bladder. However, be mindful of calories. For tea drinkers, non-citrus herbal tea may be a good choice. There are also a few coffee substitutes on the market that may be worth a try. Examples of refreshing low-acid fruits that won't irritate your bladder are apricots, papaya, pears, and watermelon.

Although there's no precise scientific evidence, it's generally recommended that women should drink 8 to 9 ½ cups of fluids per day and men about 12 cups. This includes all fluids (tea, coffee, fruit juices, liquor, etc.), and not just water. The amount you need to drink is affected by things like activity level, climate, and body weight. We'll cover this topic in more detail when we discuss the importance of staying hydrated.

Some women try to drink less fluid in order to decrease leakage, but this isn't a good idea. You should avoid restricting your fluid intake because it can be irritating to the bladder. This may lead to more leakage, and it can also place you at risk of getting a bladder infection. If you don't drink enough fluids, your urine may have an unpleasant odor and be dark-colored, like apple cider. Normal urine should have a clear to light yellow color, like pale lemonade.

Constipation exacerbates urinary incontinence. If you have a full rectum, it can push on your bladder and cause urgency and leakage. In a nutshell, aim to consume 25-35g of fiber per day. We'll address constipation in detail in Chapter 10.

Pelvic Floor Muscle Exercises for Bladder Health

Regular exercise of the pelvic floor muscles helps one to build strength, endurance, and coordination. Performing the exercises incorrectly by "bearing down" can actually worsen urinary incontinence (UI). It's best to learn to perform the exercises in a relaxed position. Start by doing the exercise lying down and gradually progress to performing them in sitting and then standing.

Pelvic floor exercises are sometimes called "Kegels." They are named after Dr. Arnold Kegel, a gynecologist who advocated the use of pelvic floor muscle contractions after pregnancy to decrease urinary incontinence. There are certain cues you can use to learn how to correctly contract your pelvic floor muscles. Women can imagine they are trying to stop their flow of urine. Alternatively, people can pretend they are trying to hold back gas in a crowded elevator.

Recall that there are fast twitch and slow twitch muscle fibers. To strengthen your pelvic floor muscles, you should perform the following two types of contractions. Try to perform 10 repetitions of each, three times per day for a total of 30 repetitions. If you so desire, you can perform up to 80 reps per day of each type of exercise.

1. **Quick contractions**: Perform a 2-second-long pelvic floor muscle contraction hold followed by a 2-3 second rest to

strengthen the fast twitch fibers. While breathing out, contract your pelvic floor muscles and hold for 2 seconds. Take in a diaphragmatic (belly) breath and repeat the pelvic floor muscle contraction when you exhale.

2. **Endurance holds**: Perform a 10-second-long pelvic floor muscle contraction hold followed by a 10 second rest to strengthen the slow twitch muscle fibers. Pull your pelvic floor muscles up and in and hold the contraction for 10 seconds (or as close to 10 seconds as you can get). Then relax for 10 seconds. Make sure that you keep breathing while you perform the Kegel. If you feel like you are holding your breath, you can count out loud while you are holding the contraction. It's easiest to start performing pelvic floor muscle exercises by lying down with your knees bent. You can support your knees with pillows. Avoid straining or using muscles other than your pelvic floor. Once you're proficient at performing the exercises, try them sitting and then standing. These positions are more challenging because of the effects of gravity pulling on the pelvic floor muscles.

Remember, make sure to relax your body (buttocks, belly, and inner thigh muscles) and don't hold your breath while contracting the muscles. Don't strain (try too hard) or bear down (bulge your private parts outwards). For the short contractions (quick flicks), you can coordinate your breathing with your pelvic floor contraction by blowing out or exhaling while you contract your pelvic floor muscles.

It's helpful to prevent wear and tear on your pelvic floor muscles as you age. One way you can do this is by performing a "pelvic brace" (also referred to as "The Knack"). A pelvic brace helps reduce leakage associated with stress UI. It involves contracting the transverse abdominis muscle (in the region of your umbilicus) at the same time as your pelvic floor muscles. Perform a pelvic brace by contracting your pelvic floor muscles (pull your pelvic floor muscles up and in). At the same time, pull in your belly button like you're zipping up a tight pair of pants. Do a pelvic brace before you cough, sneeze, or lift. I often say to my patients, "Squeeze before you sneeze."

To figure out how many times per day you are toileting, you can complete a bladder diary. It has columns for time of day, what you have eaten/drank, volume of urine (how much you have voided), level of urgency, and leakage. Later in this chapter, we will take a close look at the concept of bladder retraining, including how to complete a bladder diary.

If you feel like you're losing sleep from toileting too often during the night, there are several steps you can take. First, stop drinking fluids two to three hours before bedtime and avoid drinking caffeine at dinner. Several hours before bedtime, lie in a recliner or bed such that your feet are raised higher than your heart. Then pump your feet/ankles up and down for a minute or two. Sometimes, fluid accumulates in the feet, ankles, and lower legs during the course of the day. Ankle pumps help to push the fluid from your lower legs and feet back to your heart and then to be processed by the kidneys. This will make your last trip to the bathroom before you go to sleep more effective.

If You Feel Like You Need Professional Help

If you have concerns, you may benefit from a formal examination by a urologist, urogynecologist, or gynecologist. Sometimes urinary urgency, frequency, and leakage can be caused by a urinary tract infection. Physicians may do testing to check bladder capacity and do urodynamic testing.

Your physician may refer you for a physical therapy evaluation. Choose a physical therapist who has completed continuing education/coursework in the areas of pelvic floor dysfunction. At our facility, therapists who treat urinary incontinence hold certificates of achievement in "Pelvic Physical Therapy" as instructed and issued by the American Physical Therapy Association.

During a physical therapy evaluation, a therapist will interview the patient and ask questions about past medical history and toileting habits. Next, an examination is performed to check skin integrity; assess pelvic floor muscle strength and endurance; check reflexes; and inspect for the presence of prolapsed ("dropped") organs. We'll take a closer look at prolapse in Chapter 8.

Physical therapists use biofeedback to evaluate and treat the muscles of the pelvic floor. Biofeedback is a very effective learning technique. It utilizes specialized equipment to enable a person to see on a computer screen how their muscles are responding to instructions. After a person becomes aware of these responses, they can learn to control them (e.g., relax tense muscles and strengthen weak muscles).

You're in Control/ Urine Control: Urge Control Techniques for a Healthy Bladder

You have an urgent desire to empty your bladder. As you pull into your driveway, you think, "Thank goodness, I made it." You trek along a short walkway and fumble to get your key out of your pocket. As you insert the key into the lock, you lose control of your urine. It soaks your underwear, and you can feel some dripping down your legs. You think to yourself, "Oh no, not again." This scenario is so common that it has its own name: key-in-the-lock syndrome.

Urge Control Techniques

Urge control techniques help a person "gain control" when they have a strong urge to urinate. There are several steps you can take to decrease urinary urgency.

1. Stop whatever you are doing and stay very still. This will help you to maintain control of your bladder. DO NOT rush to the toilet, as this may lead to inadvertent leaking.
2. Do five or six quick pelvic floor muscles contractions (Kegels with a two-second hold as described previously). These short pelvic floor muscle contractions send a message to your bladder to relax and hold urine.
3. Relax, take a deep diaphragmatic (belly) breath, and let it out slowly. Diaphragmatic breathing is discussed in detail below.
4. Use distraction techniques to help the urge pass. For example, you can think about your to-do list, your favorite vacation spot, your family, count backwards by 3's from 100, or say the alphabet backwards.
5. Keep your thoughts positive. Example: "I'm not going to let my bladder control me."
6. Some find it helpful to apply firm pressure to their crotch area. You can do this with your hand or by sitting on a firm surface with a rolled-up towel pressed against your crotch.
7. If the urge returns, repeat the above steps until the urge subsides and you regain control. At that point, walk at a normal pace to the bathroom.

How to Perform Diaphragmatic Breathing to Control Urinary Urgency

Start by lying on your back or in a chair in a relaxed position. Place one hand on your chest and the other on your abdomen. Relax your jaw by placing your tongue on the roof of your mouth and keeping your teeth slightly apart. Try to focus on the relationship between your breathing diaphragm and the pelvic floor muscles. Take a deep breath in through your nose, letting the abdomen expand and rise while you keep your upper chest, neck and shoulders relaxed. As you breathe in, let the pelvic floor muscles relax.

As you breathe out through your mouth, allow your abdomen and chest to fall and tighten and contract the pelvic floor muscles (i.e., perform a Kegel exercise as described previously). Exhale completely. Remember to breathe slowly. Don't force your breathing. Your breaths shouldn't be deeper or faster than normal breaths, as this may cause you to experience tingling in your hands and feet from hyperventilating.

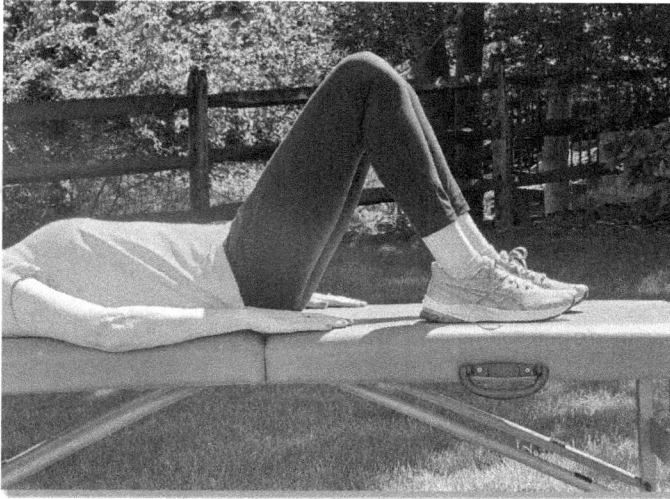

Figure 1 Diaphragmatic breathing

Keeping a Bladder Diary

To figure out how many times per day you are toileting, you can complete a bladder diary. A bladder diary helps you to understand your toileting patterns, habits, and reasons for "accidents." It can also provide possible solutions for incontinence. It is used to establish a baseline and can later be used to assess progress. To improve accuracy, fill out the log throughout the day rather than trying to recall details at the end of the day.

A bladder diary has columns for time of day, what you have eaten/drank, volume of urine (how much you have voided), level of urgency, and leakage.

Column 1: Time of Day

Column 2: Food and Fluid Intake: Write down what you ate and drank throughout the day.

Column 3: Amount of Urine Voided: Record the volume of urine. This can be approximated as small, medium, or large. You can also count how many seconds you voided. One easy way to do this is to count "One Mississippi, two Mississippi, three Mississippi…" The counting seconds method may not be ideal if you have a hesitant, start-and-stop or extremely weak stream. Thirdly, you may choose to measure the exact amount of urine with a measuring cup.

Column 4: Estimate the amount of leakage as S (small), M (medium), or L (large).

Column 5: Record whether the urge was present. 1= mild urge, 2 = moderate urge, and 3 = strong urge. Think of a strong urge as "Get out of my way. I need to go to the bathroom right away!"

Column 6: Write down what activity you were doing when you leaked, such as coughing, sneezing, laughing, walking to the bathroom with urgency, or sleeping. You may also choose to make other notes in this column.

At the bottom of the page, you can write down the number of pads used that day.

Time of Day	Amount and Type of Fluid/Food Intake	Amount Voided	Amount of Leakage	Was the Urge Present? (Mild, Moderate, Strong)	Activity with leakage/ other comments
12:00AM					
1:00					
2:00					
3:00					
4:00					
5:00					
6:00					
7:00					
8:00					
9:00					
10:00					
11:00					
12:00PM					
1:00					
2:00					
3:00					
4:00					
5:00					
6:00					
7:00					
8:00					
9:00					
10:00					
11:00					

Number of pads used: _____

Bladder Retraining Program

Complete the bladder diary for three days. Then count up how many ounces of fluids you drank, how many times you voided, and how often you leaked. What were you doing when you leaked? After incorporating the treatment strategies described above and performing the pelvic floor muscle home exercise program for a month, complete the bladder diary again to assess your progress.

If you feel like you are constantly running to the bathroom, you can use a technique called bladder retraining. This behavioral technique retrains your bladder to return to a more normal and convenient pattern of urinating. It has been found to be helpful for people with urinary urgency, leakage, and increased frequency of toileting during daytime and/or nighttime hours. It involves gradually lengthening the period of time between voids so that you increase your bladder capacity.

With bladder retraining, you follow a schedule of urinating (voluntarily emptying your bladder). The act of toileting is paired with a neutral third party, which in this case is a clock. Instead of your "bossy" bladder running the show, the clock will decide when you should use the toilet.

How to perform bladder retraining: when you wake up for the day, go to the bathroom and completely empty your bladder. Your voiding schedule will begin upon getting out of bed and will end at bedtime. That is, the schedule is for daytime hours only.

Pick a time interval that you think you can manage *without* leaking. You can look at the results of your bladder diary to help you pick an interval. For example, let's say you decide to try urinating every 2 hours. Follow this interval as closely as possible. The important part of retraining is that you practice telling your bladder when to empty and when to hold. I would rather you pick a shorter interval at first and not leak than to pick a longer time interval but leak urine.

Go to the toilet at the scheduled time even if you don't feel the need to urinate. The amount you void is not important. It doesn't matter if you void a small or large amount. Just relax and make sure not to strain while urinating.

If you need to urinate before the scheduled time, use the urge delay techniques described above. If you have to interrupt the schedule, try to get back on schedule at the assigned time for the next void.

Once you can manage 2 hours, bump up the time interval to 2.5 hours. Gradually increase the time interval as tolerated. This will slowly increase your bladder capacity. Your goal is to go 3-4 hours between urinating.

If you're sick, don't worry about the retraining program that day. Just try to get back on the program the next day. Don't be discouraged if you are influenced by fatigue, feeling nervous, cold weather, the sound of running water, or if you're about to start your menstrual period. Be patient and stick with the program. To be successful, your urges need to be suppressed on a consistent basis.

Chapter 8

Don't Let it All Hang Down: Pelvic Organ Prolapse

*E*mma Mae Hart pauses while lifting an eight-pound dumbbell at the gym. The
familiar, uncomfortable pressure in the area of her private parts is back again.
*Lately, in fact, it feels like more than just pressure. The other night, when she looked
"down there" with a mirror, she was pretty sure some tissue was "hanging out." She
is growing increasingly worried that she might need surgery if she doesn't take steps to
correct the problem soon. She recalls that when her mother was in her seventies, she
needed surgery to "lift" her bladder back up.*

A support structure composed of muscles, ligaments, and skin in
and around a woman's vagina holds her pelvic organs and tissues in place.
Think of it as a hammock which helps hold up organs such as the
bladder, bowels, and uterus. Parts of this support network may weaken,
deteriorate, get stretched out, or tear, leading to a common condition
called prolapse.

If the bladder, uterus, or bowels shift and drop downwards, it may
cause a bulging of the vaginal wall out of the vaginal opening. Anterior
vaginal wall prolapses, or cystocele, is a bulging of the bladder (the front
of the vagina bulges out due to pressure from a "dropped bladder").
Posterior vaginal wall prolapse, also called a rectocele, is a bulging of the
rectum. That is, the back wall of the vagina bulges out from the vaginal
opening due to pressure from the rectum. It is most noticeable if a person
is straining, such as when trying to push out a bowel movement. The
vaginal wall can also bulge out due to dropping of the uterus. If you have
a uterine prolapse, you may feel your cervix, which feels similar to the tip
of your nose, at your vaginal opening. Men can get a pelvic organ

66

prolapse as well. The rectum may drop down, with the bulge occurring from the anus. Women can have a rectal prolapse too.

Prolapse can cause an uncomfortable heavy feeling in your private region, especially with prolonged standing. Some liken it to the sensation of having a ping pong ball between their legs. The heavy feeling often goes away if you lie down. Some women may feel a mass bulging out of their vagina. Prolapse can affect sexual intercourse, as well as the ability to urinate or defecate. For example, it may make it difficult to pass urine or have a bowel movement. In some, prolapse can cause constipation. It may also result in stress urinary incontinence (leakage with coughing, sneezing, laughing, jumping, etc.). It's possible to have a prolapse without experiencing any symptoms. Without medical intervention, a prolapse can worsen and may eventually require surgical intervention.

Common factors that may cause a prolapse include the following:

- Childbirth: Vaginal delivery of large babies can increase the risk. Long, difficult deliveries can also contribute. The more babies born vaginally, the higher the risk.
- Menopause: When estrogen levels decrease, support structures may become weaker.
- Hysterectomy: The uterus is removed during a hysterectomy. Since the uterus provides support at the top of the vagina, a hysterectomy may cause the top of the vagina to gradually fall down towards the vaginal opening.
- Age: Risk increases as you get older.
- Obesity: Extra pounds increase risk.
- Strenuous physical activity: If your career involved heavy lifting or strenuous activity, this may increase your risk for prolapse.
- Prior pelvic surgery
- Radiation to the pelvic area
- Chronic constipation (pushing and straining)

- Chronic cough (places pressure on pelvic organs)
- Having family members with prolapse
- Smoking

Prolapse can make it difficult to get your urine out. Or you may be able to start the stream but then be unable to completely empty your bladder. Why does this happen? Prolapse may cause a "kink" in the urethra (the tubing through which your urine flows). There are several things you can do if you have difficulty voiding.

Steps to take if you have trouble completely emptying your bladder:

1. Relax. Take a few diaphragmatic breaths to allow your pelvic floor muscles and sphincter muscles to relax and release your urine.
2. Perform a few quick pelvic floor contractions as described previously. Sometimes, it helps to contract in order to be able to relax and let out the urine.
3. Double voiding: With this technique, a person voids urine, stands up, wiggles their hips and pelvis, and then sits back down to completely empty the bladder. In some instances, a person can modify this technique by remaining in a sitting position on the toilet but leaning side to side to "unkink" the tubing.
4. Bending forward: Void as much urine as you can. Then bend forward at the hips and knees and slowly reach down and touch your toes (if you can). Sit back up and repeat two more times. This puts a gentle pressure on your bladder and facilitates complete emptying of the bladder.

You can take steps to decrease your risk of prolapse and strengthen your pelvic floor. Pelvic floor muscle exercises as described previously in Chapter 7 will help to build muscle strength and endurance. If you are overweight, try to lose the extra pounds. Avoid constipation by eating a healthy, high-fiber diet, and drinking plenty of water. If possible, avoid heavy lifting. If you can't avoid lifting, learn to use proper lifting strategies as described in Chapter 14. In addition, try to quit smoking.

Low pressure fitness (LPF) is a movement approach that facilitates core strengthening, normalization and coordination of pelvic floor muscle tone, and neurodynamic/myofascial mobility. I am a Level 2 LPF instructor, and I have witnessed first-hand how integrating low pressure fitness concepts with traditional pelvic floor treatments leads to successful outcomes for my patients with prolapse, urinary incontinence, core weakness, and constipation. LPF is a movement approach which utilizes hypopressive breathing, a type of vacuum breath which originated hundreds of years ago as part of yoga (Uddiyana Bhanda). By focusing on diaphragmatic and lateral ribcage breathing, hypopressive breathing creates an abdominal vacuum which decreases pressure in the abdomen and pelvic girdle. You can learn more about LPF at www.lpf-usa.com.

Chapter 9

A Day in the Life of Your Bowels

Alexa Hayworth glances at the clock on her bathroom wall. Her job interview at a prestigious accounting firm is in 45 minutes, but it's a 25-minute drive to get there. She knows she should already be on the road. But instead, she is sitting on what she refers to as "the throne." It is a familiar scenario to her. Although she spends a lot of time on the toilet, she doesn't have much to show for it. She has great difficulty getting her stools out. She is constipated with a capital C. Her mother tells her she should see a specialist. She just never seems to get around to it.

Alfred Whitley figures he's been having bowel problems for at least twenty years. He first noticed he was constipated after suffering a small stroke when he was sixty. He took an early retirement and spent a lot of time watching TV. His doctor prescribed numerous medications the last few years. Alfred isn't even sure what they are all for. But one thing he does know: they make his constipation worse. He spends many hours of the day preoccupied with his bowels. In fact, he wonders if he is becoming obsessed with his gut. Sometimes, he misses going to church or out with the guys because he is (fruitlessly) sitting on the toilet. Boy, what he would give to defecate like he used to without putting so much thought and effort into it.

Flatulence fascinates youngsters. From bothersome gas to unwelcome constipation, many adults are consumed with thoughts of their gut as well.

The bowel is the last part of your digestive system. After the food you eat passes through your mouth, esophagus, stomach, and small intestines, it enters your bowel (also called large intestines or colon). The colon is basically a five-foot long tube that allows the food that can't be used by the body to be disposed of. Water and most nutrients are absorbed in your small intestines. However, water and some nutrients (electrolytes) are also absorbed from the large intestines.

Stool is formed in the large intestines. Peristalsis, which are contractions of the involuntary muscles (muscles that are not under your conscious control) within the intestinal walls, help to move the stool along. By the time it reaches the last section of bowel, called the sigmoid colon, it has lost much of its water content. Just before you have a bowel movement, the stool enters the last 4 to 6 inches of the colon, known as the rectum. When the rectum fills with stool, there is an increase in intra-rectal pressure. A message is sent to the brain via nerves that a bowel movement is ready to be expelled.

When the rectal wall is stretched by stool, it signals the internal sphincter muscle to allow the stool to pass into the anal canal. Whereas the internal sphincter muscle is not under conscious control, the external sphincter muscle is. That is, the external sphincter allows us to make the conscious decision to "hold it in." That way, a person can delay the bowel movement until he or she can reach a toilet.

The Bristol Stool Chart, developed by Dr. Ken Heaton of Bristol, England, categorizes the consistency of stools into seven types.[1]

Type 1: Small, hard lumps
Type 2: Lumpy, sausage-shaped
Type 3: Shaped like a sausage, but with cracks on the surface
Type 4: Shaped like a sausage or snake; smooth and soft
Type 5: Soft blobs, but with clear cut edges
Type 6: Mushy; fluffy pieces with ragged edges
Type 7: Liquid

Type 3 or 4 stool is ideal since it can be easily passed without being too watery. People with Type 1 and 2 stools tend to be constipated, whereas those with Types 5, 6, and 7 may be more apt to have diarrhea.

Take a look at your bowel movement the next time you go. What type of stool do you have?

The rectal anal inhibiting reflex is an automatic reflex of the intrinsic sphincter muscle. It's able to distinguish between liquid, solid, and gas. Let's suppose that you catch a stomach bug. It's worth noting that your body can't hold in diarrhea, the same way you can't decide to hold in vomit. Your body knows that the body must expel whatever has made you ill. Some people with constipation suffer from "bypass diarrhea." In this case, the loose water stool is able to slip past through the tiny openings in the hardened stool in the rectum. Since the body thinks it's diarrhea, it slips out of the body and can result in fecal incontinence/staining of the underwear.

Chapter 10

Constipation 101

Let's check back in with Alexa Hayworth, who we met in the last chapter when she was having difficulty evacuating her bowels before an interview with a prestigious accounting firm.

Alexa rushed out of her apartment and into her car. If she speeds, she can make it to her interview on time. She pushes down on the gas pedal and floors it through the intersection as the light changes from yellow to red. She glances in her rearview mirror and cringes. A police car pulls out of a side street and flips on its emergency lights. Now she is definitely going to miss her interview.

What happens if the stool moves too quickly through the intestines and not enough water is taken out? You get diarrhea. This can be caused by infections, contaminated food or water, or sensitivity to certain foods. For example, lactose intolerance may cause diarrhea.

On the flip side, what occurs if the stool moves slowly through the colon and too much water is removed? The stool becomes hard and difficult to eliminate. The result is constipation.

Many people suffer from constipation at some point in their lives. It can cause abdominal pain and discomfort. It can cause people to strain trying to pass their stool. It may prevent all or a portion of a bowel movement from being passed.

Do you strain to empty your bowels or feel like you can't completely empty them? Do you need to insert one of your fingers into your vagina (women) or rectal opening to assist with evacuating stool? Have you ever had somewhere to go, but got delayed because of trouble passing a bowel movement? Has it made you late for work or a social engagement?

Constipation can interrupt peoples' daily routines, leading to worry and frustration.

If you suffer from chronic constipation, you're not alone. It's estimated to affect 20-30% of the population.[1] Constipation is responsible for 2.5 million physician visits in the United States each year.

People who are constipated have difficulty passing their stools. They tend to have fewer than three bowel movements per week. Stools may be hard, making them difficult to pass. As you age, the number of bowel movements you normally have may decrease due to being less active, drinking less fluids, and eating less fiber.

Constipation may be the result of several different factors. One common cause is delaying bowel movements. A person can "put off" defecating by voluntarily contracting their external sphincter muscle. This causes the urge to pass stool to subside, which makes later attempts more difficult.

Another common cause of constipation is not drinking enough fluids. Water and other liquids make bowel movements softer and easier to pass. Laxative abuse can also lead to constipation because it decreases the bowel's ability to function properly, leading people who take them to grow dependent on them. Imbalances in the diet (too much sugar and animal fat) may lead to increased difficulty in passing stools. Constipation may also stem from medications, especially pain medicines, antidepressants, iron supplements, and tranquilizers. Low thyroid hormone levels can also cause constipation. Neurological diseases such as Parkinson's, stroke, multiple sclerosis, and spinal cord injuries may play a role. Constipation can be an early sign of colon cancer.

Have you ever experienced hemorrhoids? If you have, you probably wish you hadn't. They are swollen veins located in the rectum or at the anus. Discomfort from hemorrhoids can lead to spasming of the anal sphincter, which can disrupt bowel movements. Pregnant women may complain of constipation, which is thought to be related to hormonal changes or the pressure of the fetus on the intestines. Lack of activity, whether from bedrest or decreased exercise or walking can lead to constipation. Changes in bowel habits should always be reported to your physician.

Most people in Western society need more bulk in their diet in the form of fiber. Typical dietary recommendation for fiber is between 25-35 grams per day. Fiber helps by softening the stool and adding bulk, which makes it easier for the stool to pass. Soluble fiber attracts water and slows digestion down. Examples of soluble fiber include nuts, seeds, beans, lentils, peas, and oat bran. Insoluble fiber adds bulk and weight to stool. Examples include nuts, fruits, wheat bran, whole wheat, and brown rice. When adding fiber to your diet, it is important to drink plenty of fluids. If you are uncertain about your particular fiber needs, you should discuss them with your physician, pharmacist, or nutritionist.

Some experience a bloated feeling and have increased gas when adding fiber to their diet. However, this should pass within a few weeks. It's important to avoid regular use of laxatives and enemas as they decrease the bowel's ability to function. Next, we'll look at ways to manage constipation.

Managing Constipation

Since Alexa misses her interview with the accounting firm, she drives instead to a local pharmacy and heads straight to the aisle for people with bowel problems. She feels dizzy from the number of choices. What should she buy? Which are safe, healthy choices? She doesn't want to take one that she can become dependent on. One of her friends recently visited a physical therapist who specializes in constipation. She underwent biofeedback training and learned a special bowel massage. She decides it is time she tried physical therapy too.

You feel like your "pipes are clogged" and you'd love to clear out your gut. You hotfoot it over to the local pharmacy. As you walk down the appropriate aisle, you become overwhelmed by the choices. Each one promises relief. What are the different options? Here's a simple explanation of some of the items people utilize to deal with constipation. It's not an endorsement of the different types but rather just an explanation.

- Osmotic laxatives increase the water content of the colon. An example of an osmotic laxative is MiraLAX, which has an active ingredient of polyethylene glycol.
- Stimulant laxatives work by causing contractions in the intestines to facilitate moving the stool along. Examples include castor oil, Dulcolax, and Senokot. At one time, it was believed that they could lead to dependence. That is, once people start using them, they may begin to rely on them in order to have a bowel movement. Now, research shows that this may not be the case. It may be best to use these under the direction of a physician.
- Stool softeners prevent excessive loss of moisture from the stool, which keeps them from becoming hard. They help you avoid straining with bowel movements. Prolonged use of stool softeners may contribute to an electrolyte imbalance. They usually take about 24 to 48 hours to see effects. An example is Colace.
- Flaxseed oil is a mild stool softener. Some physicians recommend people take one capsule of flax seed oil each day to help stay regular. It can be obtained at health food stores or some grocery stores.
- Suppositories: If you have constipation, your doctor may recommend a suppository. Glycerin suppositories tend to be gentler than bisacodyl.
- Enemas are used to put liquid directly into the rectum to facilitate defecation. If you are allowed to use enemas, you may decide to try using warm water without medication.

- Fiber increases the water content of the colon. Add it to your diet slowly since it may cause gas and bloating. It helps people whether they leak stool (fecal incontinence) or have trouble with constipation. Fiber works by bulking the stool and keeping it firm yet making the movement soft and easy to pass. It aids in keeping moisture within the stool, helping to prevent diarrhea or hard stools. Although fiber makes the bowels work more regularly, it isn't a laxative. Please refer to the previous chapter for more information about fiber.
- Lubricants, such as mineral oil, slick the gut so that bowel movements can pass through more easily. They take about 6 to 8 hours to work. Do not take mineral oil with food, as it can interfere with absorption of nutrients. If you regularly take mineral oil with your meals, you could be at risk for developing deficiencies in vitamins A, D, E, and K.
- Osmotic cathartics (saline laxatives), such as Milk of Magnesia and Fleet Enemas, work by keeping water in the intestines. This allows for easier passage of stool.
- Bulk-forming agents make stools softer by absorbing water in the intestines. They take 12 hours to 3 days to see results. Examples include FiberCon, Metamucil, and Citrucel. It's possible that they may affect the absorption of some medications.

Some examples of foods that aid defecation include wheat bran, prunes, coffee, and beans. Foods that have a high fiber content tend to be helpful for moving bowels. These include:

- Cooked split peas, 1 cup   16.0g
- Lentils, 1 cup cooked   15.0g
- Pinto beans, ¾ cup   10.4g
- Avocado, medium   10.0g

- Kidney beans, ¾ cup   9.3g
- Raspberries, 1 cup   8.0g
- Pear   6.0g
- Whole grain spaghetti, 1 cup, cooked 6.0g
- Barley, 1 cup, cooked   6.0g
- Red delicious apple   5.0g
- Orange, medium   4.0g
- Banana, 1 medium   3.8g
- Almonds, 1 ounce   3.5g
- Carrots, ½ cup   3.2g
- Blueberries, 1 cup   3.0g
- Broccoli, ½ cup   2.8g
- Cauliflower, ½ cup   2.6g
- Oatmeal, 1 oz.   2.5g
- Whole wheat toast   2.0g
- Baked potato with skin   2.0g
- Corn, ½ cup   1.9g
- Wild rice, ½ cup, cooked   1.5g
- Popcorn, air popped, 1 cup   1.0g
- Lettuce, ½ cup   0.9g

The United States Department of Agriculture Agricultural Research Service has a food composition database called the USDA National Nutrient Database for Standard Reference Legacy Release. It allows people to look up the nutrient content of thousands of foods.[1]

Isolated fibers do not necessarily give us the health benefits of intact fibers (the kind that occur naturally in whole foods). Many studies have linked high fiber consumption with health benefits such as lowering cholesterol, aiding digestion, and reducing the risk of heart disease. Isolated fibers have not been shown to produce the same benefits.

Isolated ("functional") fibers are added to foods by manufacturers in order to boost the number of grams of fiber they can claim on the packaging. To find out if the fiber in your food is intact or isolated, check the ingredients. Some examples of isolated fibers include inulin ("chicory root"), maltodextrin, methylcellulose, and polydextrose. Beware of the fiber in the following fortified foods: ice cream, yogurt, white bread, juice, and fiber/energy bars. Highly refined foods such as these which boast a high fiber content most likely include isolated fibers. Bottom line: to get natural, intact fiber in your diet, eat vegetables, fruits, whole grains, legumes, nuts, and seeds. This way, you'll get the benefit not only of the fiber, but also the vitamins and nutrients they contain as well.

Intestinal Massage

Intestinal massage loosens hardened stool, releases adhesions, reduces inflammation, and can help restore mobility. It involves performing slow, circular massage movements along the path of normal intestinal mobility. Exercise caution, for the massage may result in loose stools, diarrhea, or multiple bowel movements immediately following the techniques or later in the day.

1. Lie semi-reclined in a bed propped up with pillows or in a recliner. You may wish to put a pillow under your knees for comfort.
2. Place one hand on top of the other and put them on the front of your right hip bone, located just below the right side of your abdomen. You will be using your hands to massage along the path of your large intestines.
3. Use both hands together to make slow, rhythmic clockwise circular motions (like the letter "C") as they travel upwards along the right side of your abdomen (your ascending colon), until they reach the bottom of your right rib cage.

4. Now continue to use your hands to massage with slow, rhythmic clockwise circular motions (more letter "C's") as they travel across the top of your abdomen (your transverse colon), from right to left until they reach your left rib cage.

5. Shift the direction of your hands so that they travel downwards from the left rib cage to the left hip bone (along the descending colon) and continue massaging in clockwise circular motions as you create the letter "C" with your hands.

6. Continue the bowel massage and follow along the last part of your large intestines.

7. Repeat approximately 10 times.

This massage may be performed any time of the day. Many people prefer to do it when they wake up or just before bedtime.

If you need further instructions or demonstration, ask your physician to refer you to a physical therapist or nurse who specializes in treating constipation.

Tips to Help you "GO"

- Try to go at the same time each day to promote a regular bowel schedule.

- Go after eating to take advantage of the gastrocolic reflex, which stimulates your bowels.

- Take your time and try to de-stress/avoid rushing,

- Drink 6-8 cups of fluids per day. A glass of prune juice tends to have a laxative effect, possibly due to its magnesium salts.

- Eat prunes. Yes, your mother was correct. Prunes have a laxative effect due to their high fiber content and magnesium salts.

- Hot fluids may help stimulate the bowels. If you drink coffee or tea, try moving your bowels after drinking. Even hot water may help some people develop the urge to defecate.
- Eat fiber-rich foods.
- Exercise and activity promote moving the bowels.
- Try a simple recipe such as the following to promote bowel regularity: mix one cup of applesauce (it can be sweetened or unsweetened), one cup of prune juice (it can be regular or light), and one cup of unprocessed wheat bran or oat bran. Some of my patients prefer to leave it in the refrigerator, while others prefer freezing small portions into ice cube trays. If you leave it refrigerated, mix one tablespoon of the mixture with 6-8 ounces of water or juice (apple or prune). You may increase to several tablespoons as tolerated. If you choose to freeze it, defrost a portion and mix with 6-8 ounces of water or juice (apple or prune).

If you continue having difficulties, consider visiting a gastroenterologist (doctor who specializes in the bowels).

Proper Toileting Technique to Promote Bowel Evacuation

Practice this whenever you are on the toilet and have the urge to evacuate your bowels.

- Sit on the toilet and place your feet flat on a foot stool (no tippy toes). Some people prefer to use the "Squatty Potty," though any foot stool will do. Bend slightly forward at the waist. Make sure to bend forward from your hips, rather than curling your trunk forward. Don't hunch your shoulder and upper back. You should have a slight arch in your lower back. This position creates the optimal anorectal angle for easier passage of stool. It also helps the puborectalis muscle (one of your pelvic floor muscles) to lengthen and relax, which also facilitates defecation. If the puborectalis is contracted, it will inhibit the bowel movement from being released.

- Take a low deep breath in through your nose, such that your belly pushes down towards your thighs.
- Briefly make your belly hard (tense your abdominal muscles).
- Slowly exhale through your mouth as if you are blowing up a balloon.
- Repeat this numerous times.
- Be patient for 10-15 minutes.
- If nothing happens after 10-15 minutes, get up and try again later.
- Don't strain or bear down on your rectum. NO breath holding!

In the outpatient physical therapy facility where I work, we routinely address constipation in our patients suffering from urinary incontinence because it is a possible cause of bladder problems. When the rectum is full of stool, it may push on the bladder, leading to urinary urgency, frequency, and leakage. Therefore, addressing constipation can lessen bladder problems.

We also treat patients with dyssynergic defecation. People with this condition have difficulty sensing stool in their bowels or have trouble emptying their bowels. Using a wonderful learning tool called biofeedback, we help correct improper contraction of the anal sphincter and pelvic floor muscles during defecation. Electrodes are placed on the skin, near the anal opening. Alternatively, an internal (anal) sensor may be used. The biofeedback unit shows the electrical activity of the pelvic floor muscles, allowing the patient to learn how to relax the muscles and thereby facilitate bowel movement.

In conclusion, don't just sit back and let life pass you by as you sit on the "throne." There are proactive steps you can take to regain control of your bowels.

Chapter 11

Staying Hydrated

As a physical therapist specializing in urinary incontinence, the topic of hydration frequently comes up. Sometimes, my patients avoid drinking fluids in hopes of having less urinary urgency and leakage. Unfortunately, limiting fluid intake may irritate your bladder and place you at increased risk for urinary tract infections. On the other hand, some people drink so much that it's no small wonder they're always "running for the bathroom." A person with a dry mouth may sip fluids all day long. What's an ideal amount to drink?

Most people have heard that you should drink eight 8-ounce cups of water (that's about two liters) per day. It may surprise you to know that this is not based on scientific evidence. After an extensive review of literature, Heinz Valtin from the Department of Physiology at Dartmouth University found no evidence to support this notion.[1]

As you can imagine, recommendations for daily fluid intake vary. It's generally recommended that women should drink 8 to 9 ½ cups of fluids per day and men about 12 cups.[1] Others recommend 6 to 8 cups of fluids for women. Another common recommendation is 1.6 ounces per 2.2 pounds of body weight (50 ml per kg). That's total fluids: water, coffee, tea, soda, juice, etc. However, this is a general guideline for a sedentary person in a temperate climate. A person who is exercising or laboring, especially in a hot region, may require more fluids. Likewise, people with certain medical conditions may be instructed by their physician how many ounces of fluids to drink each day. In practical terms, the more high-salt foods you eat, the more water you need to drink.

People may check the color of their urine to see if they're drinking enough. Urine is usually clear to pale in color, like a light-yellow lemonade. If your urine is dark, like apple cider, consider increasing your fluid intake.

What if your urine has an odor? This can be due to the foods you eat, the classic example being asparagus. Certain medications or an infection can also create a smell. It can also be an indication that you may not be drinking enough fluids. If you have a concern, check with your physician.

Can you drink too much? Yes! It can result in a potentially life-threatening condition called water intoxication (also known as hyperhydration, water poisoning, or water toxemia). Initially, symptoms include nausea, confusion, headache, and vomiting. In later stages, seizures, coma, and even death can occur.

The excessive water causes an electrolyte imbalance. Specifically, the sodium concentration in the blood goes down (known as hyponatremia). This causes water to move into the cells. When this occurs in the brain, the cells have a limited ability to expand due to the skull. This results in the neurological symptoms outlined above.

Although this type of death is rare, it can occur. Perhaps the most well-known case occurred in Sacramento, California in 2007.[2] Twenty-eight-year-old Jennifer Strange died tragically after drinking about two gallons of water as part of a radio contest called "Hold Your Wee for a Wii." Several hours after consuming the water, she complained of a terrible headache and passed away.

Athletes are also at risk. In 2014, seventeen-year-old Zyrees Oliver drank two gallons of water and two gallons of Gatorade at football practice in Douglasville, Georgia.[3] He collapsed and was found to have massive brain swelling from over-hydration. Tragically, he was placed on life support and later died.

Play it safe by following the guidelines above or the recommendations of your physician to stay safely hydrated.

Part III: Keeping Your Framework Healthy:
A Guide to Healthy Muscles, Joints, and Bones

Chapter 12

Bone Health: Keeping Your Framework Strong

*L*isa *DeWitt doesn't think people get osteoporosis until they reach their eighties. At least, that's what she believed until last week, when she tripped on the corner of her comforter while making her bed. Even though she landed on a carpeted surface, she broke her left wrist in two places. Her doctor sent her for bone mineral density testing and diagnosed her with osteoporosis. She was astounded! After all, she had just turned 59 years old. She wished she'd learned the risk factors for brittle bones sooner. Then she could have been more proactive about maintaining her bone health.*

Osteoporosis is a condition in which bones become weak and fragile, making them more susceptible to fractures. Sometimes people refer to it as brittle bone disease. Osteoporosis means "porous bones," indicating there is a loss of bone tissue. Bones can break from minor falls or even sneezing.

Osteoporosis is most commonly seen in the spine, hips, and wrists. Some people think that bones are not alive. However, this could not be further from the truth. Inside each bone is a veritable factory: new bone tissue is being created and old tissue is being absorbed.

Children and young people create more bone cells than they lose. Peak bone mass—the highest bone density—occurs between ages 18 and 25. If you have high peak bone mass, you are less likely to develop osteoporosis later in life. As you approach middle age, you begin losing more bone tissue than you make. If you lose too much bone or make too little bone, osteopenia (lower than normal bone mass) and eventually osteoporosis may result.

If you have osteoporosis, you're not alone. Approximately 10 million Americans have the condition and another 34 million are at risk for getting it.[1] It's estimated that one in two women and one in four men over the age of fifty will fracture a bone due to osteoporosis.[2] Osteoporosis and the fractures that result from it are expensive. In fact, it's estimated that it will cost more than 25 billion dollars by 2025.[3]

You can't feel your bones getting weaker. That's how osteoporosis sneaks up on people. As your bones become thinner, they don't cause pain. However, it can cause you to lose height and have a stooped over posture (kyphosis) from compression fractures, leading to back pain.

Often, the first sign of osteoporosis occurs when a person falls and breaks a bone. Fractures can be extremely serious. They may lead to pain and disability, preventing you from doing the things you enjoy. In fact, twenty percent of senior citizens who break a hip die from complications of the fracture.[1] People who can't regain independence following a hip fracture may have to live in a nursing home.

You can improve your bone density at any age, but it's crucial to build strong bones when you're younger. That gives you a buffer, so that as you get older and lose bone, you are less likely to develop osteoporosis. Women may lose up to 20 percent of their bone density in the first five to seven years following menopause, when estrogen levels fall.[1] Men are also at risk, though later in life. When testosterone levels fall, this can increase bone loss.

So, what can you do about it? First, learn the risk factors for developing osteoporosis. Some can be controlled, while others can't. Risk factors that you can't control include age (the older you are, the higher the risk), gender (80% of people with osteoporosis are female), family history (heredity and genetics play a major role), and race/ethnicity (Caucasians, Asians and Hispanics are more likely to develop the disease). Being small and thin, menopause, various medical conditions (for example, emphysema/lung disease, diabetes, and eating disorders), and certain medications (like steroids and some cancer medications) place you at risk for developing osteoporosis. Risk factors you can control include:

- **Diet:** The foods we eat, including certain vitamins and minerals, affect our bone tissue.
- **Smoking:** Smoking makes it harder for bones to absorb calcium, which is essential to bone health. The chemicals in cigarettes harm bone cells. Also, smoking may impair estrogen from protecting a woman's bones.
- **Lack of exercise:** People who are inactive are at high risk for developing osteoporosis. To stay dense, bones need to "work." They do this by handling impact, such as when your heel touches the ground when you walk.
- **Drinking alcohol:** Two drinks per day is generally considered safe for bone health. More than that reduces bone formation. In addition, if you're "tipsy," your risk of falling increases.

Osteoporosis is diagnosed with a bone mineral density (BMD) test. This test is also called dual x-ray absorptiometry (DEXA). According to the Bone Health and Osteoporosis Foundation (BHOF), the following should have a BMD test:

- Women age 65 or older
- Postmenopausal women under age 65 with risk factors for osteoporosis
- Men age 70 or older
- Men age 50-69 with risk factors for osteoporosis
- Women going through menopause with certain risk factors
- Adults who break a bone after age 50
- Adults with certain medical conditions or taking certain medications

- Postmenopausal women who have stopped taking estrogen therapy or hormone therapy

If you have osteoporosis, your doctor may decide to place you on medication. Antiresorptive medications slow the breakdown of bone and maintain or improve bone density. These include bisphosphonates, calcitonin, estrogen agonists/antagonists, and estrogen therapy/hormone replacement. Anabolic medications, such as parathyroid hormone, help to build bone more quickly. Discuss the pros and cons of each type with your physician and pharmacist.

Now, let's explore ways to improve bone health through diet, exercise, utilizing good posture and body mechanics (i.e., moving safely), and improving your balance.

Eating for Bone Health

Everyone's heard the old saying, "You are what you eat." But did you know that what you eat directly impacts your skeleton? In order to have healthy bones, a body requires calcium, vitamin D, protein, and a healthy diet including fruits and vegetables. Let's explore each of these in greater detail.

Calcium

Calcium is essential for life. It helps us build strong bones when we're young, and it helps us to maintain healthy bones as we age. The vast majority of calcium—over 99%--can be found in our bones and teeth. It also plays an important role in bodily functions such as allowing nerves to send messages throughout our bodies, muscle contractions, and blood clotting.

Every day, we lose calcium in our sweat, urine, and bowel movements. We can't make our own calcium. That means the only way to get it is through our diet. If we don't get enough calcium to meet our needs, our body must take it from our bones. That can lead to osteopenia and osteoporosis.

The Bone Health and Osteoporosis Foundation (BHOF) recommends that women 50 years of age and older and men age 71 and older consume 1200 mg of calcium each day. Women ages 19 to 49 and men ages 19 to 71 should get 1,000 mg per day. The body can only absorb 500-600 mg of calcium at a time, so make sure you don't take all 1200 mg at once. For example, if you take a 500 mg calcium supplement with a glass of milk (300 mg), you won't absorb all 800 mg. The safe upper daily limit for calcium is thought to be 2,000-2,500 mg. Higher levels may increase the risk of kidney stones.

You can calculate the amount of calcium you get each day by using the nutrition facts label on the foods you eat. For example, if the label says the food contains 30% of the daily value of calcium, that usually means it contains 300 mg. Likewise, if it says 15%, that means 150 mg. There are some exceptions, such as when the food is from another country which has different nutrition guidelines. Note that typically, the average person gets about 250 mg of calcium without even trying because the mineral is present in smaller amounts in our diet. So, if you add up the amount of calcium consumed using nutrition facts labels, add 250 mg to your total. The BHOF provides a comprehensive list of calcium rich foods on its website, including the number of milligrams of calcium per serving. The International Osteoporosis Foundation (IOF) has a similar list on its website. These tools can give you a general idea of how much calcium is present in the foods you eat. For example, a cup of milk has 290 to 300 mg of calcium, while a cup of yogurt has 240 to 400 mg. Do you want to feel good about eating ice cream? A half cup has 90 to 100 mg of calcium. Three ounces of canned salmon with bones has 170 to 210 mg. Another good source is ½ cup of cooked kale (90 to 100 mg) or turnip greens (11 to 125 mg).

You can increase the calcium content of food by adding powdered milk into pancake and cookie batter or bread dough. You can also add it into puddings, custard, or cocoa. A tablespoon of nonfat powdered milk has approximately 50 mg of calcium.

If you find that you need a calcium supplement, try to find one that has the USP (United States Pharmacopeia) symbol or states that it is purified. Most calcium supplements should be taken with food because eating produces stomach acid, which helps your body to absorb calcium. Calcium citrate supplements absorb well with or without food.

Certain foods, such as beans and wheat bran, contain phytates. Phytates block absorption of calcium. So, for example, if you eat wheat bran cereal with milk, your body can't absorb all the calcium from the milk. Likewise, foods that contain oxalates, such as spinach and rhubarb, make it difficult for the body to absorb the calcium in these foods. Although they are part of a healthy diet, they cannot be relied upon to provide calcium.

Vitamin D

According to BHOF, people ages 50 and over should have 800-1,000 IU (international units) of vitamin D each day. Those ages 19 to 49 should get 400-800 IU of Vitamin D daily. According to the National Academy of Medicine and National Institutes of Health the safe upper limit of vitamin D is 4,000 IU per day for most adults. Your physician may determine that you need more than the recommended daily allowance. Make sure to follow your physician's guidelines.

We get vitamin D from sunlight, food, and supplements. Our skin makes vitamin D from ultraviolet rays. The amount our body makes varies with proximity to the equator (the closer to the equator, the more Vitamin D we make), season (summer more than winter), and time of day (more vitamin D when the sun's rays are stronger). People with lighter skin make more vitamin D than those with darker pigmentation. Those who live north of the line between Atlanta and Los Angeles are too far north for their skin to make enough vitamin D during the winter.

It's difficult to get enough vitamin D from food. It's present in fatty fish (salmon, tuna, mackerel), liver, and egg yolks. It's added to some foods, like milk and some brands of cereal and orange juice. Since it's challenging to get enough Vitamin D from food, a supplement may be necessary. Studies have shown that vitamin D2 (ergocalciferol) supplements are as effective as vitamin D3 (cholecalciferol). If you have osteoporosis, a simple blood test can tell you your vitamin D level.

Other vitamins and minerals, such as magnesium, potassium, vitamin K, and vitamin C are all important to bone health. If you eat a healthy, well-balanced diet, you are most likely getting enough of these vitamins and minerals. If not, consider taking multivitamins or supplements. Your physician can assist you in making this decision.

Protein

In general, for optimal bone health, women should strive to eat about 60 grams of protein daily. Men should aim for 80 grams. A diet that is too high in protein, especially animal protein, may cause a loss of calcium through the kidneys. Check with a dietician if you desire specific guidelines for protein intake.

Salt

Eating too much salt can cause bone loss, since an excess of salt causes the body to lose calcium. Consuming 2,400 mg or less salt per day should not be harmful to bones. Try to avoid processed foods, which are typically high in salt. Put the saltshaker away and look for healthier alternatives for seasoning your food, such as herbs. More to come on salt when we discuss blood pressure.

Exercise for Bone Health

Henry Cooper hates the way he hunches over when he walks. He used to be able to straighten up with effort, but now it seems like his back is permanently stuck in a bent-forward position. His doctor sent him for x-rays last week. She said the stooped-over posture is due to compression fractures in his spine from osteoporosis. She discussed nutrition with him and referred him to physical therapy, stating, "It's never too late to learn how to exercise."

Exercise is an important component of bone health. Bones get stronger and denser when you make them "work." Work for bones means making them handle impact. This can be our own body weight, or it could be in the form of resistance, like weights or exercise bands. Weight-bearing exercises and muscle-strengthening exercises are the most important.

Weight-bearing exercises are those in which one moves against gravity while in an upright position. When I am standing up, my feet are bearing weight on the ground. Likewise, if I do a push-up, my hands are bearing weight on the ground. Weight-bearing exercises can be high or low impact. Examples of high impact exercises include jogging, running, jumping rope, soccer, tennis, basketball, gymnastics, dancing, and hiking. Generally, low-impact exercises are safer for patients with osteoporosis. Examples include fast walking outside or on a treadmill; using elliptical or stair-stepping machines; and low impact aerobics.

Strive to perform weight-bearing exercises for thirty minutes most days of the week. In terms of bone health (as opposed to a cardio workout), it doesn't matter if the thirty minutes are all together or broken up into three ten-minute sessions. If you have trouble fitting it into a busy schedule, get creative. For example, try taking the stairs (at least for several floors) instead of an elevator. Park farther away from stores or from your workplace to encourage walking. Use a health app on your cell phone that tracks steps. Set a daily goal to motivate you to get more steps in.

Muscle-strengthening exercises, or resistance exercises, are those in which you move your body, a weight, or a resistance band against gravity. For optimal results, they should be done 2 to 3 days per week. Yoga, Pilates, and using weight-lifting machines are examples of muscle strengthening exercises. People with osteoporosis need to avoid exercises in which they bend forward at the spine (flexion), because these can increase the risk of a spinal fracture. This means you should avoid exercises such as toe touches and sit-ups. Forward bent postures in Yoga and Pilates are also risky and not recommended. People who have broken spinal bones in the past due to osteoporosis should also avoid rapid twisting motions and heavy lifting.

Resistance exercises should target the large muscle groups of the body. Aim to perform 1-2 sets of 8-12 repetitions (reps). If you can't do eight in a row, the weight or resistance band is probably too heavy. If you can easily do more than 12 reps, the weight may be too light. If you have osteoporosis, it may be better to do 10-15 repetitions with a lighter weight to avoid straining or injuring yourself.

People often ask if biking and swimming are good for your bones. Unfortunately, since they are not weight-bearing exercises, they don't help bone density. However, they have other benefits, such as cardiac conditioning. Also, cycling and swimming are gentler for people who have arthritic joint pain or fibromyalgia pain.

Balance exercises are important if you have osteoporosis. Since people with osteoporosis have fragile bones, a fall could lead to a fracture. We'll discuss balance in more depth in Chapter 18.

Sometimes as people age, they develop a forward head posture, rounded shoulders, and a curved spine. Posture exercises help to improve posture and strengthen spinal muscles. They can help to decrease the risk of spinal fractures. Stay tuned for more about posture.

Functional exercises improve how well you move during daily activities. Examples include standing up and sitting down, stair-climbing, and rising up on the toes (lifting your heels off the ground) while standing.

If you already have osteoporosis, avoid twisting your spine to the point of strain and bending forward during activities such as coughing, sneezing, vacuuming, and lifting. Also, avoid reaching too high or too far in front. For example, don't put heavy items in the back of a high cabinet or the fridge. When getting out of bed, turn to your side first rather than sitting straight up from a supine position.

A physical therapist can help create a home exercise program to build bone density, strengthen muscles, and improve balance and posture. Also, many communities offer exercise classes for bone health. The following is an exercise program that I have developed for my patients with osteoporosis and osteopenia. In the PT clinic, I modify it for each person's individual circumstances.

Osteoporosis Home Exercise Program
Building Bone Density and Muscle Strength

Walking (Weight-bearing) Program:

As described above, try to achieve 30 minutes of weight-bearing activity through walking, treadmill walking, ellipticals, or recumbent ellipticals each day. Remember, the 30 minutes does not have to be all together (it can be spread out throughout the day). If you are new to walking and exercise, start with a short walk (perhaps a few blocks out and few blocks back) and gradually increase the distance.

Research shows that use of a weighted vest while walking may improve bone density or prevent further bone loss. If you decide to try walking wearing a weighted vest, start by adding one pound. Gradually increase with an eventual goal of adding 10% of your body weight. For example, if you weigh 200 pounds, you could gradually increase the added weight of the vest to 20 pounds. The theory is that by adding weight, you are adding impact to your steps, which builds great bone density. If you have back pain, a weighted vest may not be for you. If you are uncertain, check with your physician.

Upper extremity resistive band exercises:

Bands come in different colors, representing differing amounts of resistance. Choose a band that is challenging but does not cause pain. If you are not sure, err on the side of choosing a lighter resistance.

Note: The next three exercises can be performed in hook lying (lying down with knees bent and feet flat) or standing. Performing them in hook lying may be easier at first and provides more stability to your spine. After you become proficient at performing them in either position, you may choose to do them in either hook lying or standing, depending on what you prefer and what works best for your schedule. You can even do them once during the week in hook lying and the second time in standing.

Shoulder external rotation in hook lying or standing: Lie on your back with your knees bent and your feet flat on the surface or stand. Stretch the band keeping elbows against your sides and keeping elbows at 90 degrees. Perform 2 sets x 10 repetitions, 2-3 times per week.

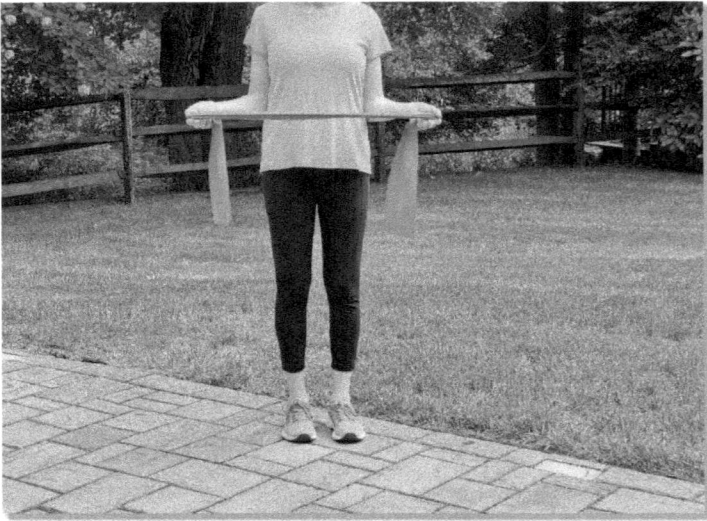

Figure 2 Shoulder external rotation

Supine horizontal abduction in hook lying or standing: Lie on your back with your knees bent and your feet flat on the surface or stand. Hold the band up towards the ceiling. Pull your arms out to the sides and gently allow your shoulder blades to squeeze together. Perform 2 sets x 10 repetitions, 2-3 times per week.

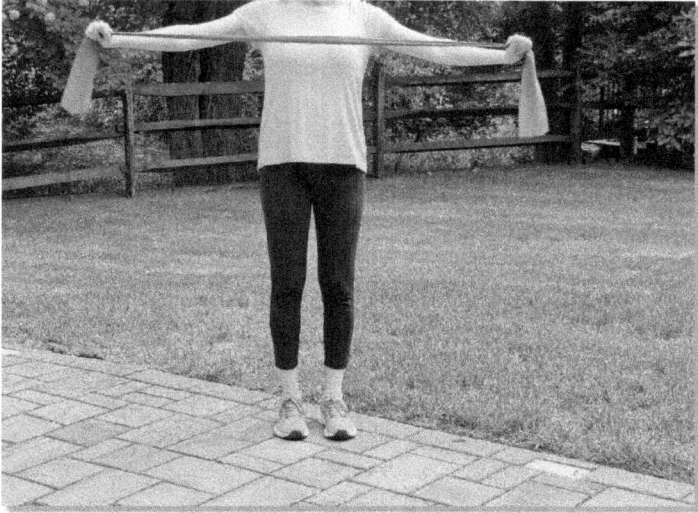

Figure 3 Shoulder horizontal abduction

PNF D2 pattern in hook lying or standing: Lie on your back with your knees bent and your feet flat on the surface or stand, holding onto one end of a resistance band in one hand by your side. With the opposite hand holding the opposite end of the band, pull the band into a diagonal direction. Act like you are drawing a sword from its scabbard by rotating at your shoulder until your thumb is facing the wall. Avoid bending your elbow. Then, slowly return toward the hip. Perform 2 sets x 10 repetitions, 2-3 times per week.

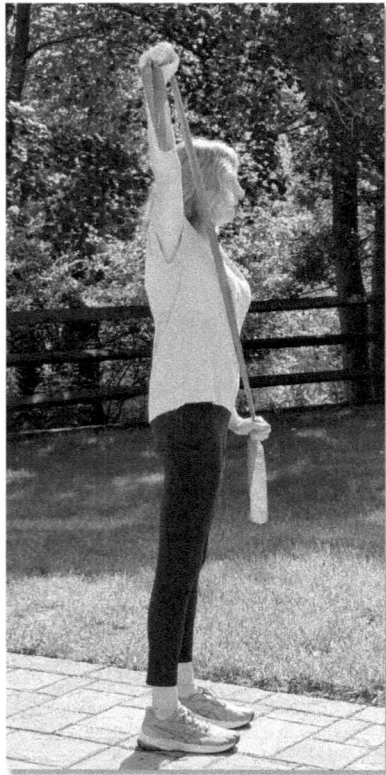

Figure 4 PNF D2 pattern

Rows with elastic band: Holding the elastic band with both hands, draw back the band as you bend your elbows. Keep your elbows near the sides of your body. Pretend like you are sliding your arms back on a tabletop, such that your forearms are parallel to the floor. Perform 2 sets x 10 repetitions, 2-3 times per week.

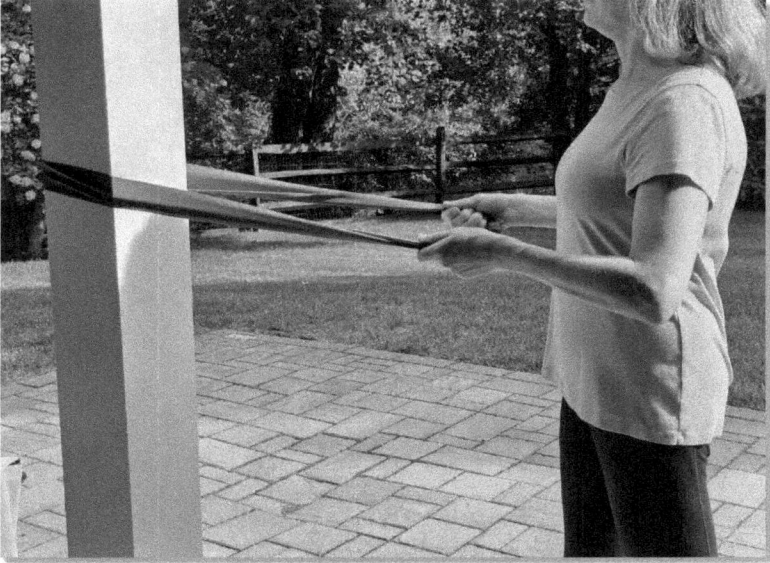

Figure 5 Rows with elastic band

Shoulder extension with elastic band: Start with a little tension in the elastic band, arms straight, about 30-45 degrees away from your body. Keeping your arms straight, bring your arms back and down towards your sides. Return to starting position. Perform 2 sets x 10 repetitions, 2-3 times per week.

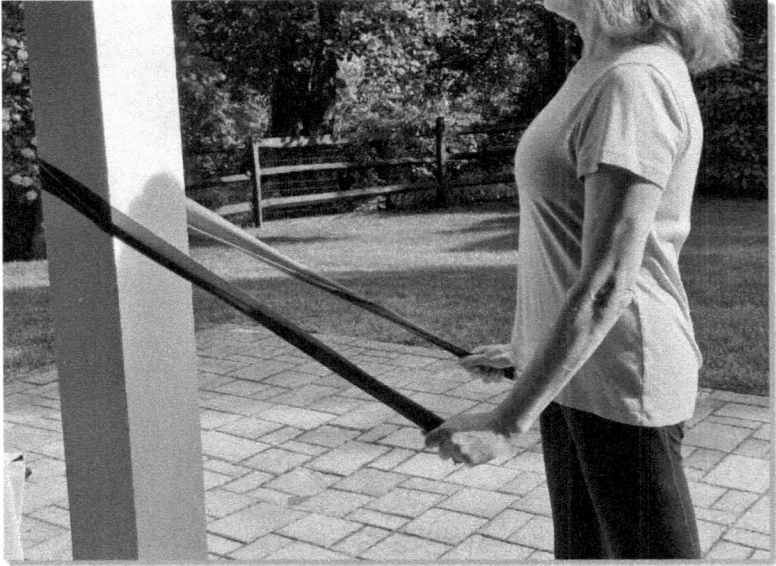

Figure 6 Shoulder extension with elastic band

Wall press-ups: Stand facing a wall and place your feet a comfortable distance away, about 18-24 inches. Place your hands on the wall with palms at shoulder height. Lean into the wall, allowing your elbows to bend. Push back out, straightening your arms. This is a modified version of a traditional floor push-up. Perform 2 sets x 10 repetitions, 2-3 times per week.

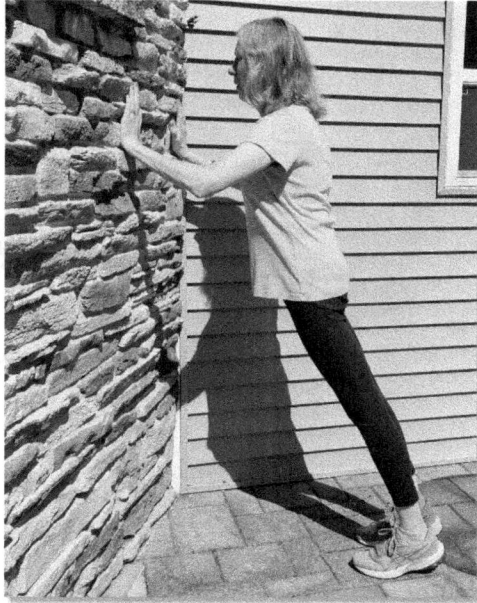

Figure 7 Wall press-ups

Quadruped alternate arm lifts: While in a crawling position on your hands and knees, slowly raise one arm out in front of you or to the side of you (whatever is more comfortable). Hold 2 seconds and repeat 10 times with the left arm, then 10 times with the right arm. If you are able, complete a second set of 10 with each arm. Bearing weight on each upper extremity promotes an increase in bone density.

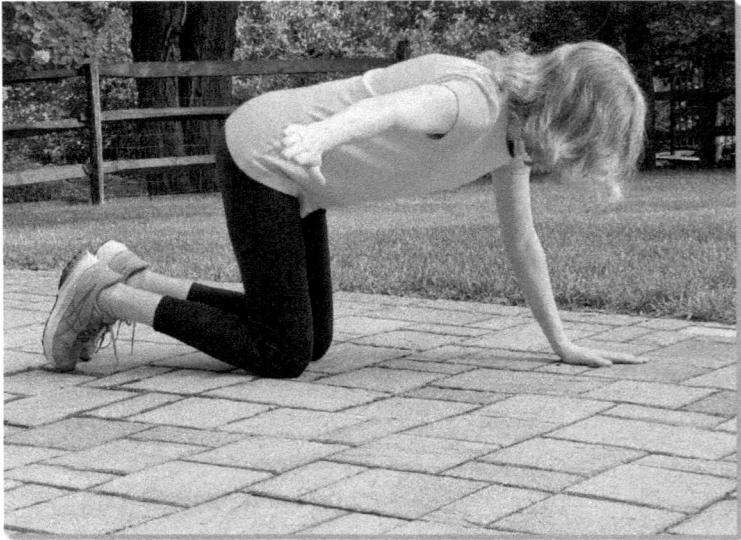

Figure 8 Quadruped alternate arm raise

Upper extremity strengthening exercises with weights

Forward raises (bilateral flexion to 90 degrees of elevation):
While standing with your arms by your side, slowly lift your arms up to
shoulder level. Hold a free weight/dumbbell in your hands if you are
able, making sure it is the appropriate weight. Repeat 2 sets x 10
repetitions, 2-3 times per week.

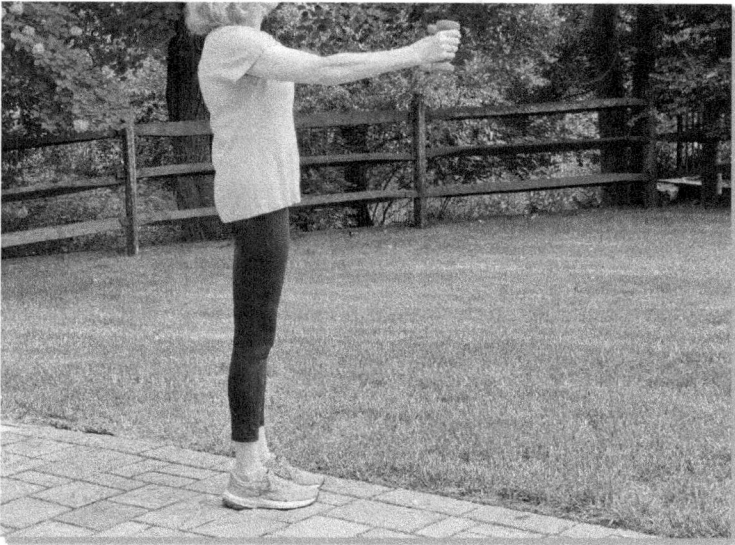

Figure 9 Forward raises

Sideways raises (bilateral abduction to 90 degrees of elevation): While holding a free weight/dumbbell in both hands and with your elbows straight, raise your arms up from your side with the palms facing downward. Lower and repeat. Repeat 2 sets x 10 repetitions, 2-3 times per week.

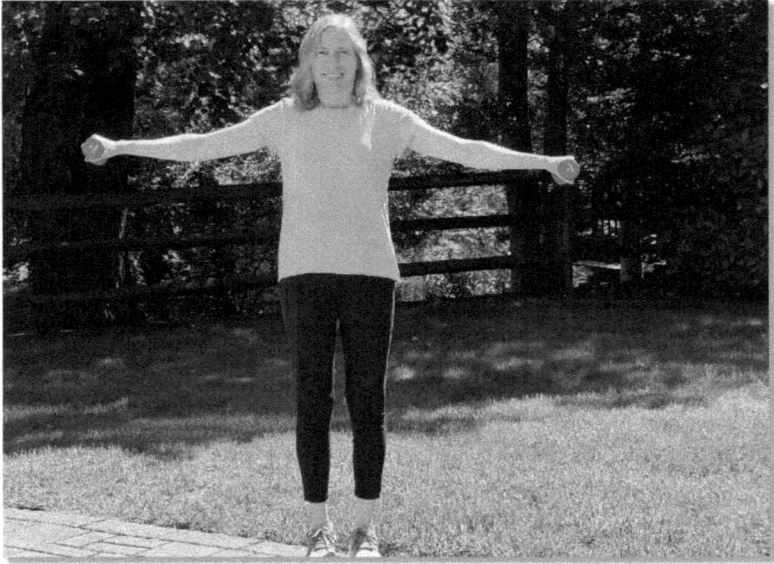

Figure 10 Sideways raises

Biceps curls: While sitting in a chair and holding a free weight/dumbbell on each thigh, lift both sides while bending at the elbows. Lower back down and repeat. Alternatively, you may perform this exercise while standing (without resting the weights on your thighs between repetitions). Repeat 2 sets x 10 repetitions, 2-3 times per week.

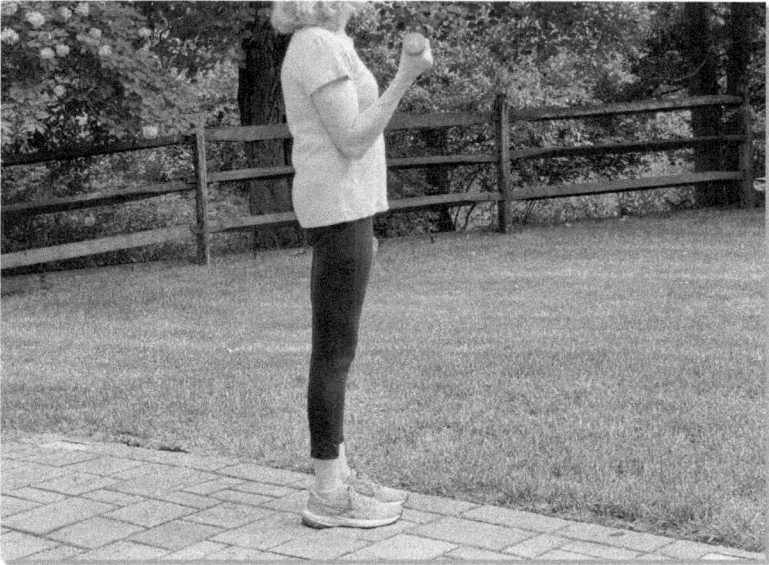

Figure 11 Biceps curls

Bent over triceps (triceps kickback extension): While standing, bend over and support yourself with one arm. With your other arm, hold a free weight/dumbbell and keep your elbow at your side with it in a bent position. Repeat 2 sets x 10 repetitions, 2-3 times per week.

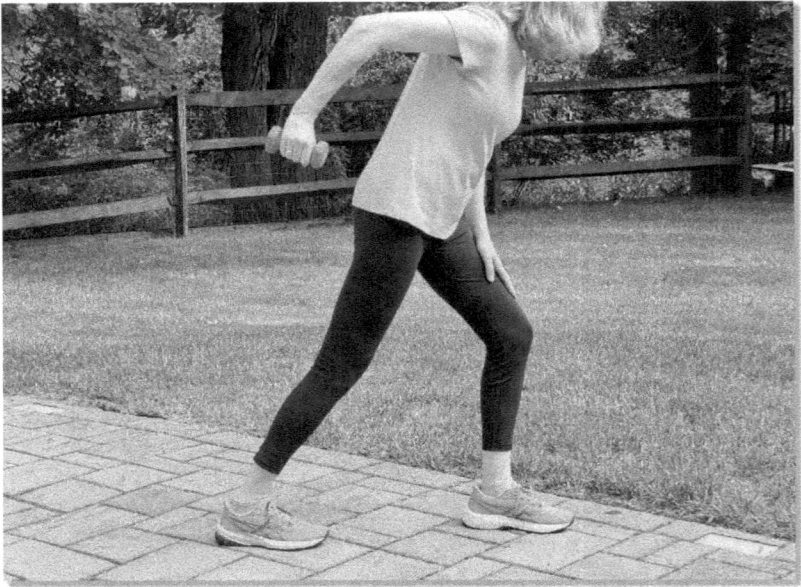

Figure 12 Bent over triceps

Lawnmower: Stand with your right arm at your right knee in a semi-squat position. Pull your right elbow back as if you are starting a lawn mower or snow blower (similar to a sawing motion). Hold a dumbbell in your hand if you are able, making sure it is the appropriate weight. Repeat 2 sets x 10 repetitions, 2-3 times per week for each upper extremity.

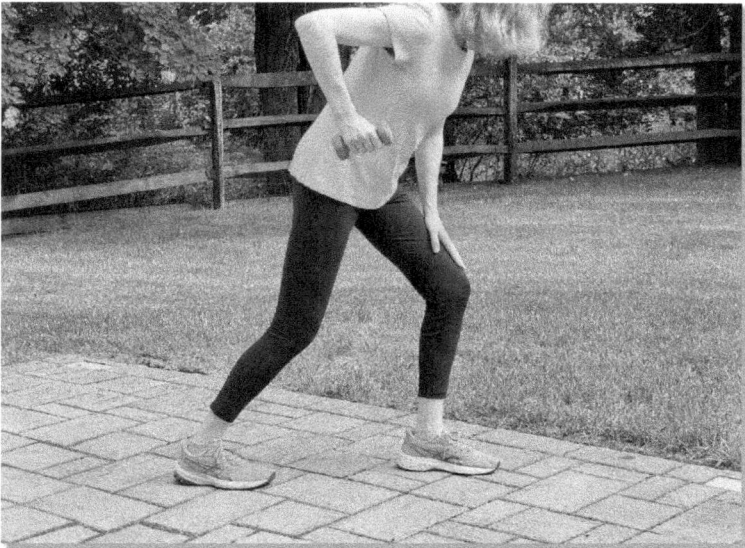

Figure 13 Lawnmower

Wrist flexion curls: While holding a small free weight/dumbbell, place your forearm on your thigh and bend your wrist up and down with your palm facing down as shown. You may support your wrist with your other hand. Alternatively, support your forearm on an armrest. Repeat 2 sets x 10 repetitions, 2-3 times per week.

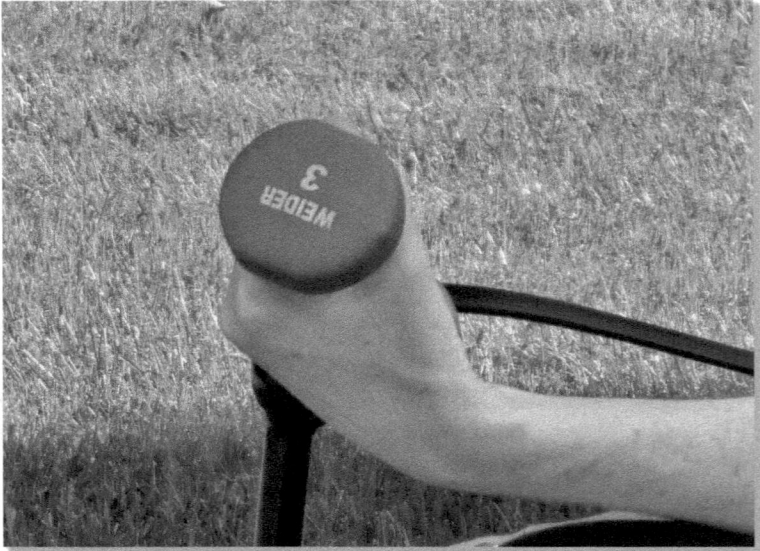

Figure 14 Wrist flexion curls

Wrist extension curls: While holding a small free weight/dumbbell, place your forearm on your thigh and bend your wrist up and down with your palm facing up as shown. You may support your wrist with your other hand. Alternatively, support your forearm on an armrest. Repeat 2 sets x 10 repetitions, 2-3 times per week.

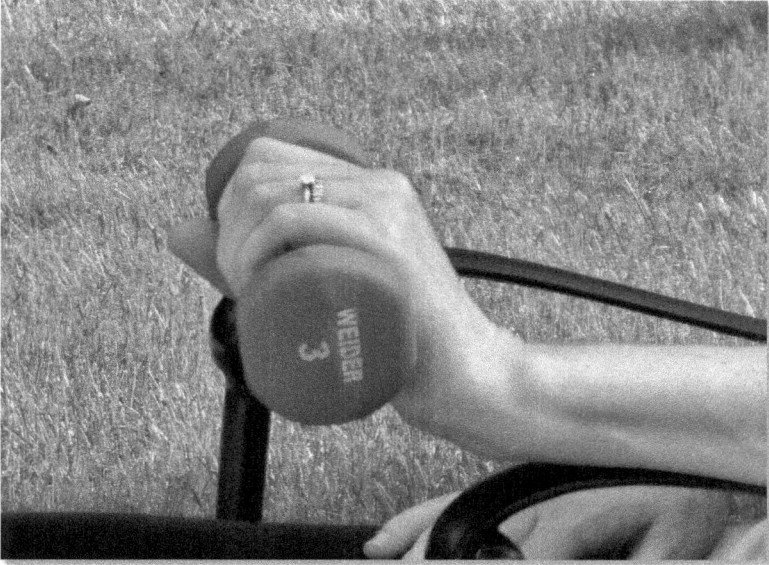

Figure 15 Wrist extension curls

Umbrella Breathing: Stand with your back against a wall or lie on your back with your knees bent up (hook lying). Inhale for 2 seconds through your nose and allow your belly to expand while your ribcage opens like an umbrella. It may be helpful to place your hands on the sides of your ribcage, so you feel the expansion laterally. Exhale for 4 seconds through your mouth. Repeat 10 times, once per day.

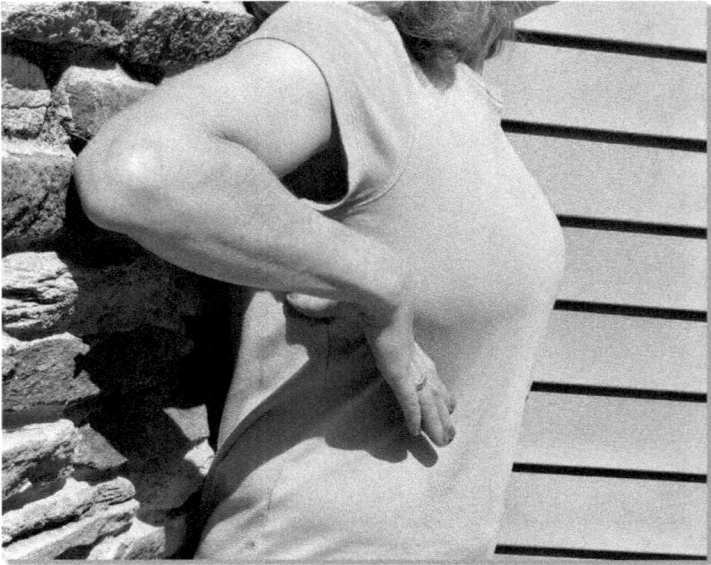

Figure 16 Umbrella breathing

Standing lower extremity strengthening and weight-bearing exercises

Standing marching (hip flexion): While standing next to a chair or countertop for support, march in place by lifting your knee up as you allow it to bend and then perform on the other side. Repeat this alternating movement. Use your arms for balance support if needed for balance and safety. Use cuff weights around your lower legs if you are able. Repeat 2 sets x 10 repetitions, 2-3 times per week.

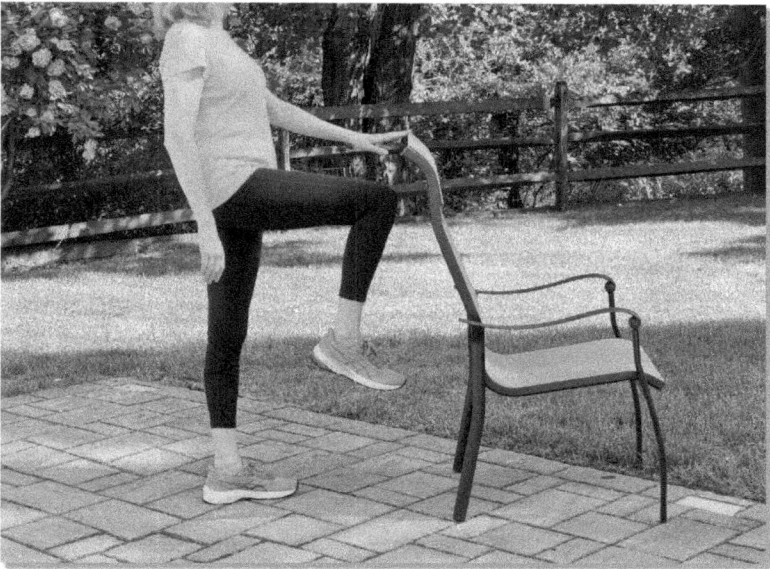

Figure 17 Standing marching (hip flexion)

Standing hip abduction: While standing next to a chair or countertop for support, raise your leg out to the side. Keep your knee straight and maintain your toes pointed forward as best as you can. Then, lower your leg back down and repeat. Use your arms for balance support if needed for balance and safety. Use cuff weights around your lower legs if you are able. Repeat 2 sets x 10 repetitions, 2-3 times per week.

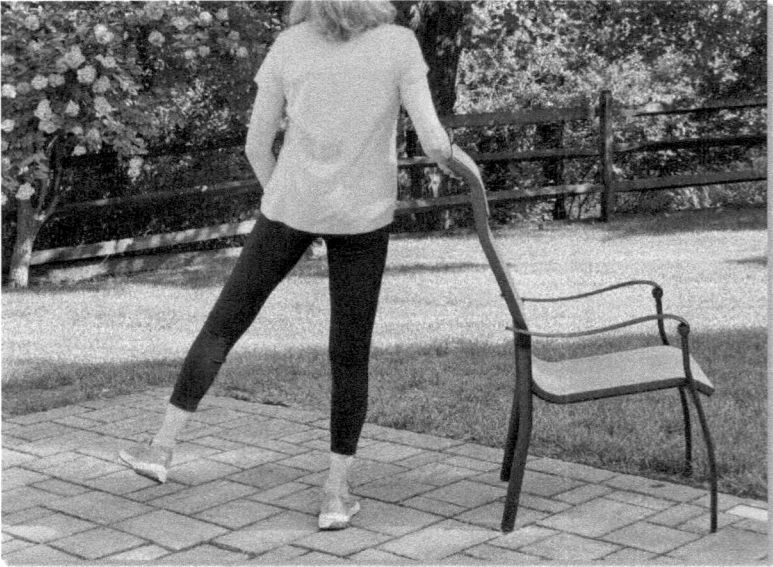

Figure 18 Standing hip abduction

Standing hip extension: While standing, stand on one leg and move your other leg in a backward direction. Do not swing your leg but rather create slow, smooth, controlled movements. Keep your trunk stable and do not arch your low back during the movement. Use your arms for balance support if needed for balance and safety. Use cuff weights around your lower legs if you are able. Repeat 2 sets x 10 repetitions, 2-3 times per week.

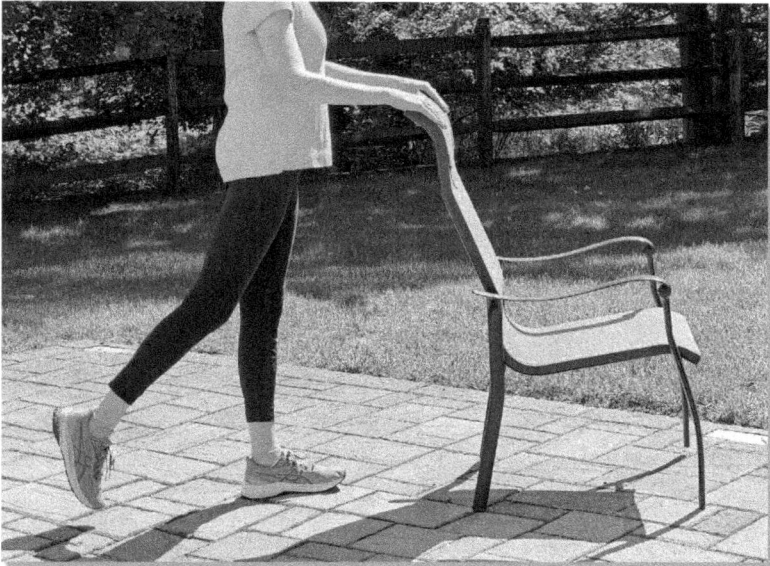

Figure 19 Standing hip extension

Mini squat: Stand with your feet shoulder width apart and toes pointed straight ahead. Next, bend your knees to approximately 30 degrees of flexion to perform a mini squat. Then, return to the original position. Pretend like you are sitting down in a chair. Your kneecaps should not come forward past your toes. Use your arms if needed for balance and safety. Repeat 2 sets x 10 repetitions, 2-3 times per week.

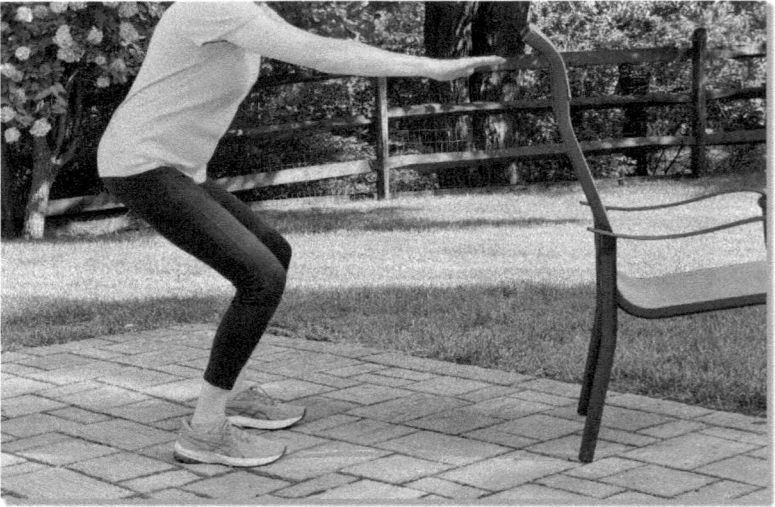

Figure 20 Mini squat

Heel and toe raise: Stand at a counter or other sturdy support surface. Rise onto your toes and hold. Then rock back onto your heels, lifting your toes. Perform in a slow, controlled manner. Use your hands on the support surface for balance if needed. Try to stay as tall as possible while performing this exercise. Repeat 2 sets x 10 repetitions, 2-3 times per week.

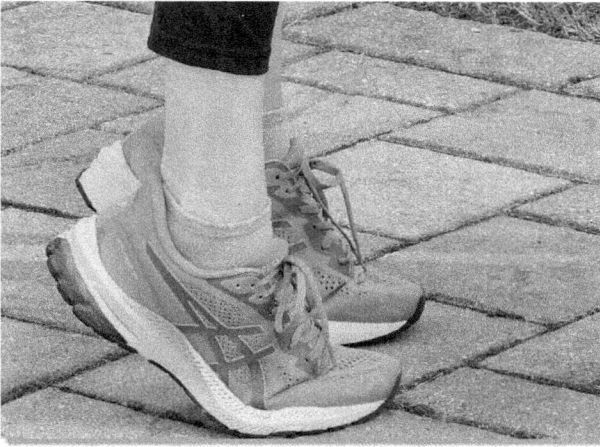

Figure 21 Heel raise

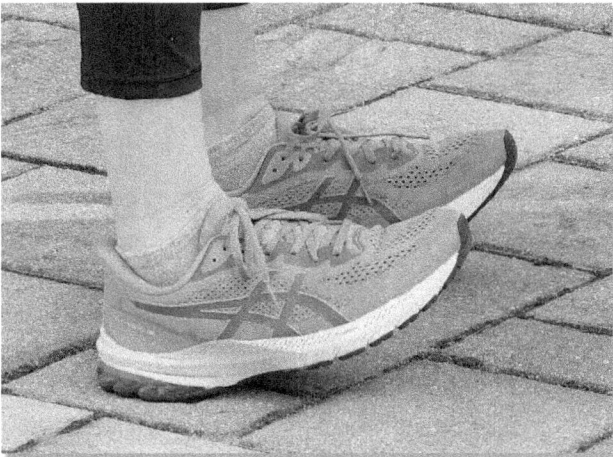

Figure 22 Toe raise

117

Single limb stance: Stand at a counter or other sturdy support surface. Lift one leg off the floor and balance on the other foot for 60 seconds. You may use light hand support as needed. Then, switch legs and balance on the other foot for 60 seconds. Research shows that balancing on a single leg for 60 seconds three times per week for at least 24 weeks builds bone density in the hip.[4]

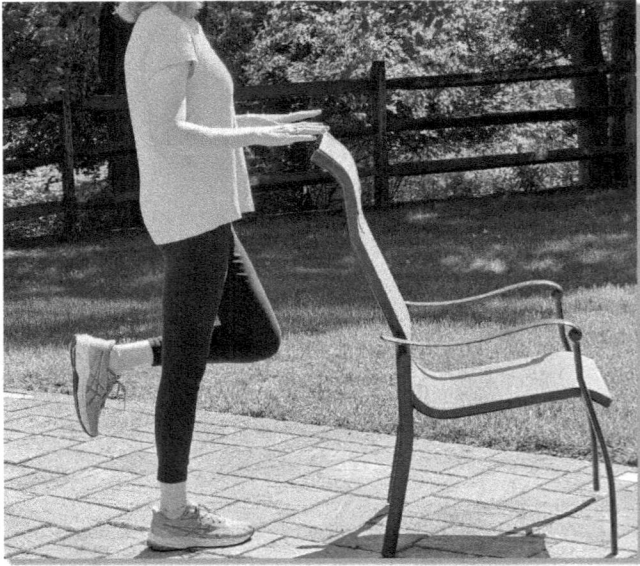

Figure 23 Single limb stance

Chapter 13

Staying Flexible: Stretching Muscles Safely

Tyrone frowns as he stares down at his feet. He hasn't been able to bend over and touch his toes since the second grade. That is more years ago than he cares to admit. Lately, his back feels stiff too. The local gym is offering a special deal on yoga classes. He decides he'll give yoga a try.

Have your muscles been tight your whole life? Do your hamstrings prevent you from reaching forward and touching your toes? Do tight calf muscles make it uncomfortable for you to bend and straighten your ankle? Or perhaps you experience a more general feeling of tightness.

There are many advantages to safely stretching your muscles. Stretching improves range of motion (how far you can move your joints) and flexibility (how easily you can move your joints). It may also decrease the risk of injuries and even improve athletic performance. Stretching allows your muscles to work more effectively by helping your joints to move through their full range of motion. This could translate into an increase in your reach during a tennis match or improvement in your golf swing. Stretching increases blood flow to the muscle, which improves circulation. Proper stretching can improve posture and create a sense of well-being. In addition, stretching tight muscles may reduce pain.

As people age, muscles, and tendons (which connect muscles to bone) may become tighter. If the muscles of the buttocks and legs become tight, they can impact your walking pattern by making your stride shorter. Tight muscles may make it difficult to perform seemingly simple activities, like tying your shoes or reaching down to pick something off the ground. If you set aside time to make stretching part of your routine, it will help your muscles age in a healthy way.

You may hear muscles referred to as agonists and antagonists. An agonist causes a movement to occur, while an antagonist produces an opposing joint torque (force) to the agonist. Agonists and antagonists often work in pairs. For example, if the biceps muscle in the front of your arm contracts to bend your elbow (agonist), the triceps muscle relaxes and lengthens (antagonist). Conversely, if the triceps muscle contracts to straighten your elbow (agonist), then the biceps muscle relaxes and lengthens (antagonist). Another common example of an agonist-antagonist pair would be the quadriceps muscle (front of your thigh) and the hamstrings (back of your thigh). When you contract your hamstrings, you bend your knees, and your quadriceps lengthen. When you contract your quadriceps and straighten your knee, your hamstrings lengthen. So, when you stretch an agonist, you shorten its antagonist.

You should gently warm up your muscles with five to ten minutes of exercise, such as walking or jogging, before you stretch. Alternatively, you can stretch after you finish your work-out. Even on days when you are not doing aerobic exercises or strength training, you can still stretch as long as you warm up with five minutes of activity first. Cold muscles can be injured if they are stretched too far or too vigorously. Think of a rubber band: a frozen rubber band may break if you try to stretch it too far. A warm rubber band, on the other hand, is supple and ready to stretch. It goes back to its original shape when you let it go.

Try to have equal flexibility from side to side, especially if you have a history of a previous injury. For example, if you stretch your left hamstrings, be sure to stretch your right hamstrings too.

Focus on major muscle groups, such as your calves, thighs, hips, lower back, neck, and shoulders. Stretch muscles and joints that you routinely use at work or play. Make sure to use proper technique. Stretching incorrectly may do more harm than good. Stretch in a slow, smooth movement without bouncing. Ballistic stretching (bouncing as you stretch) can cause injury to your muscles because the muscles may reflexively shorten (tighten) and even tear. Never force or jerk yourself into a stretch.

Hold your stretch for thirty seconds. Breathe normally as you stretch (don't hold your breath). Repeat each stretch several times as tolerated. Ideally, stretch regularly (three times per week). Gently stretch or pull just hard enough to feel an easy, gentle, stretch. When you let go of the stretch, the muscle should feel relaxed and pain-free. Stretching should never be painful.

If you don't stretch regularly, you risk losing the benefits that stretching offers. That is, if stretching has helped you to increase your range of motion, and you stop stretching, your range of motion may decrease again.

If you have a chronic problem or an injury, you may need to modify your stretching techniques. For example, if you already have a strained muscle, stretching it may further harm it. Even if you stretch regularly, you can still get injured. If you're uncertain or have health concerns, check with your physician, physical therapist, or trainer about the most appropriate way to stretch.

Consider not stretching before an intense activity, such as sprinting or track and field activities. Some research suggests that stretching before these types of events may actually decrease performance, and stretching before exercise does not reduce the risk of injury.[1]

In the upcoming chapters, we'll discuss how to stretch muscles of the spine and extremities.

Chapter 14

Back Basics for a Healthy Spine

Tyler Wilson shifts uncomfortably in his desk chair. Ever since he's driven home from vacation last week (eight hours with one brief stop for fuel), his back has been killing him. He can't sleep because he can't get comfortable no matter what position he tries, whether it be on his back, stomach, or side. His wife warns him he is taking too many ibuprofen tablets. Even though he is popping them like candy, it doesn't ease his pain. He knows it doesn't help that he's gained weight over the past few years. The extra pounds around his waist increase the strain on his lower back. If he doesn't feel better by tomorrow, he'll call his doctor.

Have you ever experienced back pain? For most people, the answer is yes. According to the National Institute for Neurological Disorders and Stroke, about 80% of the population suffers from back pain at some point in their lives.[1] At any given time, a quarter of Americans report experiencing low back pain within the past three months.[1] Low back pain is the number one cost in workers compensation payments and a leading cause of lost workdays each year.[1]

Low back injuries can cause pain, inconvenience, lost time, expense, and disability. It's a popular myth that back injuries are caused by one specific, traumatic event in a person's life. In actuality, the development of low back pain is rarely an isolated incident. Usually, it's a cumulative series of small injuries (microtrauma) that leads to larger injuries. Then one day, the "straw breaks the camel's back."

Acute low back pain lasts a few days to a few weeks. Subacute low back pain lasts four to twelve weeks. Once the pain is present for longer than twelve weeks, it's known as chronic pain. Approximately one-fifth of patients with acute low back pain go on to develop chronic pain.[1]

Understanding the Basics: Anatomy of the Spine

The spine has numerous purposes. It provides mobility and stability, protects the nerves and spinal cord, and acts as a shock absorber. The spine allows both mobility and stability. This allows us to do activities with our arms such as cooking, reaching, and lifting and with our legs such as walking, running, and climbing. The bony structure of the spinal canal protects our spinal cord, which runs through it. The discs which separate the bones of the spine (vertebrae) act as shock absorbers.

There are thirty-three vertebrae, most of which have a disc separating them. There are seven cervical vertebrae in the neck region, twelve thoracic vertebrae in the mid region of the spine (connected to the ribcage), five lumbar vertebrae (low back), five fused vertebrae of the sacrum, and four (three to five) fused bones of the coccyx (tailbone). Since the sacral vertebrae and coccyx are fused, there are approximately twenty-five moving segments.

Your spine has three important, noticeable curves: cervical lordosis (arch of the neck region), thoracic kyphosis (curve of the middle back), and lumbar lordosis (natural arch in your low back). The function of the curves is to increase the load bearing capacity of the spine and help to absorb shock. By having the curves, your spine is able to handle loads (weight applied vertically downward through the spine) ten times greater than if it were a perfectly straight column.

To understand how the spine works, you first need to know the anatomy. A spinal segment, or motion segment, includes the adjacent halves of two vertebral bones, the disc between them, the facet joints (small joints between each set of adjacent vertebrae), and the corresponding contents within the spinal canal. The supporting ligaments, muscles, blood vessels and nerves are also included. The primary function of a spinal segment is to provide motion. It also allows for weight-bearing and offers protection to the spinal cord and nerve roots. A loss or alteration of motion in the spine or any joint in the body may lead to pain.

Spinal nerves branch off the spinal cord and travel through small openings on either side of the vertebral column. The spinal nerves from the cervical region of the spine travel to your arms. Spinal nerves from the thoracic spine innervate your organs and trunk. Spinal nerves from the lumbar and sacral areas travel to your legs, allowing you to move and feel/sense.

Intervertebral discs bind vertebral bodies together, permit motion between spinal segments, and transmit shock. The outer ring of the disc, called the annulus fibrosus, resists tensile forces and confines the inner part of the disc (the nucleus pulposus). The nucleus pulposus distributes forces and acts as a ball bearing. You may have heard someone say that they "slipped a disc." This means that the disc has herniated. Most often, part of the disc material migrates backwards (posteriorly) or back and off to the side (posterolaterally). If the bulging disc presses on sensory nerve fibers, you'll feel pain or experience numbness and tingling. If it presses on motor nerve fibers, you may experience weakness in your legs. Disc herniations can be a major cause of low back pain and disability.

There are three layers of spinal muscles. These muscles contract to allow motion and provide support via muscle tone. At rest, while performing activities or lifting, they work to hold the spine as well as the whole body in an erect position.

The superficial layer includes muscles that most people are familiar with, such as trapezius (in the neck), latissimus dorsi (large muscle of the back), and gluteus maximus (buttocks). The intermediate layer includes the erector spinae, which runs the length of the spine. The deepest layer primarily involves the motion segments of the spine. One of the most important deep muscles is the multifidus. Basic functions of this muscle include backward bending, side bending, and rotating the spine. It can "turn off" after a back injury and therefore may need to be retrained.

When talking about abdominal strength, one of the buzzwords today is to have a strong "core." Your transversus abdominis (TrA) muscle is located near your umbilicus (belly button). It's the innermost flat abdominal muscle. If you pull your belly button in as if you're zipping up a tight pair of pants, you're contracting your TrA. In order to increase your core strength, you must strengthen this muscle. The muscles in your back are designed to provide stability to your spine. The muscles in your buttocks and legs should provide the power behind lifting.

The spinal ligaments restrain and limit motion of your vertebrae. They protect the facet joints and strengthen the intervertebral disc. Facet joints are important because they both guide and limit spinal motion. They also allow for weight-bearing through the spine. The principal function of the ligaments is to limit or modify movement occurring at the spinal motion segments.

Numerous factors can contribute to low back pain, such as stress, poor fitness, inadequate nutrition, and smoking. For example, stress can lead to tight, painful muscles. Poor fitness can cause weakness and poor posture. It's important to have an adequate supply of nutrients for the tissues of the body to do their jobs. There's a higher incidence of back pain in smokers. Smoking decreases the oxygen brought to the muscles. Taking steps to address these factors may help to reduce the incidence and severity of back pain.

Good Posture and Body Mechanics for a Healthy Spine

Most of us are familiar with the stereotype of the slouching teenager. When you were young, did anyone ever recommend that you walk with a book balanced on the top of your head to improve your posture?

Posture is the way you hold your body. Good posture does more than tell the world that you're self-confident. It's important to have good posture in both sitting and standing for a multitude of reasons. Poor posture can cause headaches as well as neck, back, and jaw pain. Poor head and neck posture can affect your ability to swallow. A hunched over spine can impact your ability to take a deep breath.

Poor sitting posture includes a forward head, rounded shoulders, and a slouched (rounded) spine. If a person has good sitting posture, the ears should be in line with the shoulders and hips. Picture a string pulling straight upward on your head. Good posture is your tallest position with your feet flat on the floor.

Most people like to sit at their desk to surf the web or do paperwork. Your desk should have the monitor set at or just below eye level. Your elbows, hips and knees should be bent between 90 degrees (a right angle) and 110 degrees. Try to maintain an upright posture as described above. Keep your feet flat, resting comfortably on the floor. Remember, you can adjust things like monitor height, keyboard height, seat height, and footrest height until you feel comfortable and have proper alignment of your spine. If you feel like you need more support for your lower back, you can try using a lumbar roll. You can purchase one online or make your own by rolling a towel and placing a rubber band at each end to keep it from unrolling.

It's also important to maintain a good position while driving. Sit close enough to the pedal and wheel to avoid slouching. Use a lumbar roll as needed to support your lower back. Try not to sit for long periods of time without getting up.

Sitting is the most stressful posture for our spines. If you're a couch potato or you have a job that requires you to sit for long periods of time and if you don't have spinal stenosis (a narrowing of your spinal canal), you can put your hands on your hips and bend backwards five times every 30-60 minutes. Test this motion with care, as back bends can increase pain in people with spinal stenosis. Back bends (also known as lumbar extension) help to minimize damage and maintain normal function of your discs and muscles. It's another important tool for healthy aging of your spine.

Similar to poor sitting posture, people with poor standing posture tend to have a forward head, rounded shoulders, and a slouched spine. Good standing posture means that your ears are in line with your shoulders, hips, and ankles. You should keep your head and shoulders back and your spine should have its natural curves as described previously.

When standing, try to change positions often and keep your work in a comfortable, convenient position. It may be helpful to occasionally shift your weight from one foot to the other or rest one foot up on a box or stool. If necessary, rest your back by leaning on a wall or sitting down for a few minutes. Avoid slouching and try to stand straight up, since poor posture can cause back pain. You should also avoid wearing high heels or hard soled shoes for too long, standing in one position for a prolonged period of time, standing with your knees locked, or standing bent forward with your work in a low position.

Sleeping Posture

If you already have neck, back, or joint problems, sleeping posture is extremely important. Sleep on a mattress that is comfortable for you. Make sure it's on a firm, stable foundation. A firm box spring will prevent even a soft mattress from sagging.

If you're a back-sleeper, place one or two pillows under your knees to take the strain off your low back and allow your hips to relax. If necessary, place a small towel roll in the small of your back to help you maintain the natural curve of your lower back.

If you are a side-sleeper, place a pillow under your head and another between your knees. The pillow between your knees will help to keep your low back straight, preventing strain. If you have large hips and a small waist, it may be helpful to place a small towel roll under your waist.

Lastly, place a pillow in front of your chest and rest your upper arm on it.

Being a stomach sleeper can cause neck pain. However, if you decide to sleep this way, you can place a pillow under your stomach to prevent excessive sway-back.

Don't Get Injured When Lifting: Use Good Body Mechanics

As you get older, you may not have the same strength as when you were younger. This means you're even more likely to get injured if you utilize improper lifting techniques. Part of healthy aging means being smart and using good body mechanics during lifting to avoid harming yourself.

It's natural to think you can keep lifting the heavy objects that you hoisted up when you were younger. Don't risk it! Even young people can suffer lifting injuries. As a physical therapist, I once treated a young woman who needed back surgery after pulling apart her old deck. Another needed surgery after lugging heavy pavers across his yard to build a new patio. Be wary of backyard demolition projects or jobs which involve heavy, repetitive lifting. Young people may not experience pain with heavy lifting but wear and tear are occurring. Unfortunately, pain from damage may catch up with them as they become older.

Some tips for safe lifting include:

- A planned lift is a safe lift. If the object is too heavy or awkward to lift, ask someone to help you.
- Try to get as close to the object as possible. The farther the object is from you, the more pressure you will have on your lower back. For example, a 10-pound box held two feet in front of you could increase your low back pressure by as much as 100 pounds.

- Never lift with your feet together because it can throw off your balance. Instead, have your feet shoulder width apart or stagger your stance so you have a wider base of support.
- Keep your head up and maintain the curve in your low back when lifting. You can do this by extending your back slightly to let your butt stick out. This places your back muscles in the best position to utilize their strength and prevent disc injuries.
- Bend at your hips and knees (not at your waist) when lifting.
- Keep the object close and use your leg muscles to stand upright to lift the object.
- Never bend, twist, and lift in combination. Face the object you are planning to pick up.
- Pivot (move) your feet when lifting an item from one surface to another. Make sure you position your feet and body so that you are directly facing forward to where you want to set the object.
- When lifting, pushing, or pulling, take your time and don't use a jerky motion.
- Don't strain while lifting.
- If you have a choice, push; don't pull. Pushing is much easier for your back.

The Basics: How to Tighten your "Core"

Jenna Peterson looks in the mirror and sighs. Ever since she gave birth to her children three decades ago, she'd kissed her flat tummy goodbye. Now she struggles to keep her "muffin top" tucked inside her waistband. One of her friends recently got a tummy tuck. Another suggested she take a Pilates class to tighten up her core. Jenna doesn't want to admit it, but she isn't sure what "core" means.

Having a strong core is helpful for balance, gait, reaching, athletics, and many different everyday activities. Having a strong core will help you to continue golfing, dancing, and enjoying life as you get older.

As you recall, the transverse abdominal muscle (TrA) is the deepest layer of abdominal muscles. It is an important muscle for core strength and pelvic girdle stability. The TrA muscle aids in supporting the abdominal contents and works as a team with the pelvic floor muscles (more on these in a future chapter). Regular exercise of the TrA builds muscle strength and endurance.

The TrA exercise is a low intensity "holding" contraction of the abdominal wall. The contraction creates a feeling of deep tension and drawing in of the abdomen. When you perform a TrA contraction, your lower back should be in a neutral position (not too arched and not too slouched, but rather right in the middle). Always perform the exercise at 30-40% of maximal effort. Do not strain, bear down, or bulge your abdomen as you do the exercise. If you feel the quality of your muscle contraction decline (you feel straining or bulging of the abdominal muscles), stop the exercise session.

To perform the TrA isometric exercise, start by lying down with your knees bent. Inhale by taking a deep diaphragmatic (belly) breath. Next, tighten your TrA. You can do this by pretending you are trying to zip up a tight pair of pants. This draws your naval (belly button) toward your spine without moving or tilting your pelvis. It flattens the lower and side muscles of your abdomen. If you place your fingers under your navel, you'll feel the contraction under your fingertips. Exhale as you maintain the contraction. Remember: do not bulge your belly or allow any pelvis or back movement.

Contraction of the TrA is a "building block" exercise. That is, once you can perform it correctly, it can be used in conjunction with other exercises as you work on strengthening your core.

The exercises below can help keep you strong and flexible as you get older. They're not intended to cure pre-existing back problems. If any of the exercises cause pain or worsen your existing pain, seek the advice of a physician or licensed physical therapist for guidance.

Start by performing each of these exercises 10 times, once per day. Aim to build up to 2 or 3 sets of 10 repetitions.

Lumbar Stabilization Exercises to Increase Core Strength

Transverse abdominis (see instructions above): Hold the muscle contraction at 30 to 40% of maximal effort for 5 seconds.

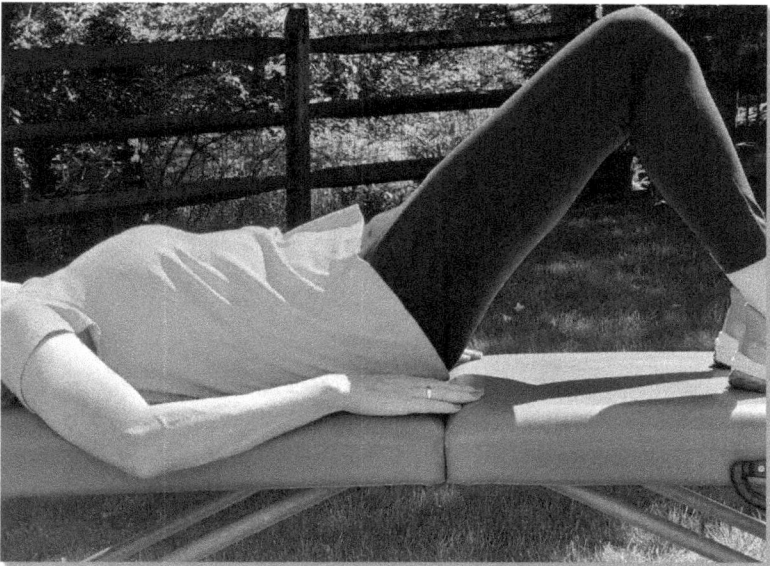

Figure 24 Transverse abdominis (TrA)

Isometric hip adduction (ball squeeze): Lie down on your back and bend your knees up so that your feet are flat on the bed (the hook lying position). Place a rolled towel, 8 to10 inch-diameter ball, or pillow between your knees. Tighten your abdominals (TrA) by drawing your stomach inward toward your spine as described above. Do not hold your breath. With your abdominals tight, squeeze the ball firmly between your knees. Hold for 3 seconds, relax, and repeat.

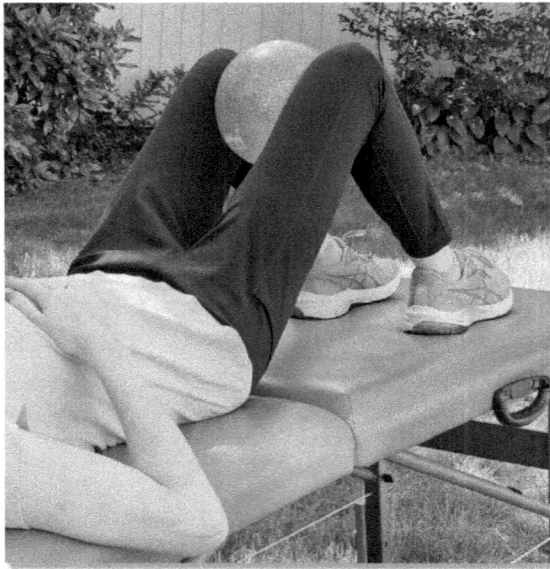

Figure 25 Isometric hip adduction (ball squeeze)

Brace-knee fall out: While lying on your back with both knees bent and your feet flat on the bed, tighten your abdominals (TrA) by drawing your stomach inward toward your spine. Do not hold your breath. With your abdominals tight, slowly lower one knee out to the side, towards the surface of the bed. Your pelvis should remain steady while your leg moves. Return to the starting position and then lower the other knee to the side. Relax and repeat.

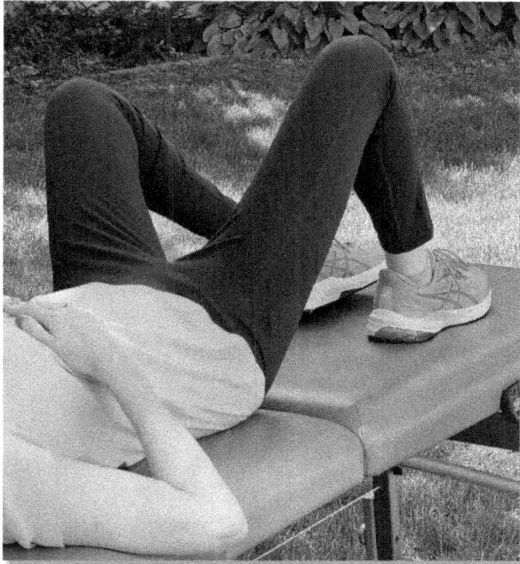

Figure 26 Brace-knee fall out

Supine hip abduction with elastic band: Lie on your back with your knees bent and your feet flat on the bed. Place an elastic resistance band around your legs, just above the knees. Tighten your abdominals (TrA) by drawing your stomach inward toward your spine. Do not hold your breath. With your abdominals tight, bring your knees apart against the resistance of the elastic band. Hold for 2 seconds and slowly bring your knees back together. Relax and repeat.

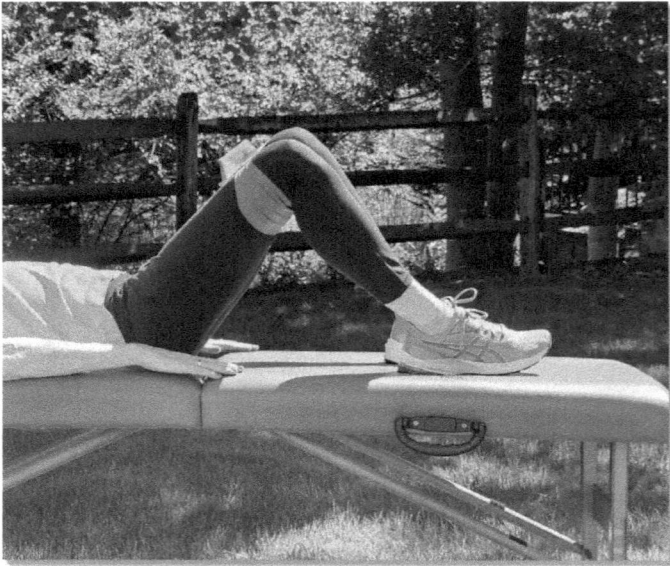

Figure 27 Supine hip abduction with elastic band

Transverse abdominis mini marches: While lying on your back with your knees bent and feet flat on the bed, tighten your abdominals (TrA) by drawing your stomach inward toward your spine. Do not hold your breath. With your abdominals tight, slowly lift one foot about six inches off the surface of the bed. Return this foot to the surface and perform with the other leg. Alternate each leg 10 times, such that you are "marching." Make sure to tighten your abdominals prior to each lift.

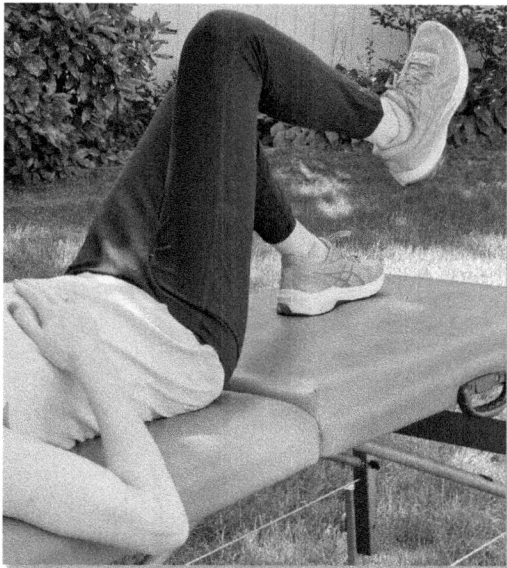

Figure 28 Transverse abdominis mini marches

Bridging: Lie on your back with your knees bent and your feet flat on the bed or mat. Tighten your lower abdominals (TrA), tighten your buttock muscles, and then raise your buttocks off the floor/bed (creating a "bridge" with your body). Hold for 3 seconds without holding your breath. Relax and repeat. Skip this exercise if you have a diagnosis of spinal stenosis, as it is considered an "extension" exercise and thus may aggravate your pain.

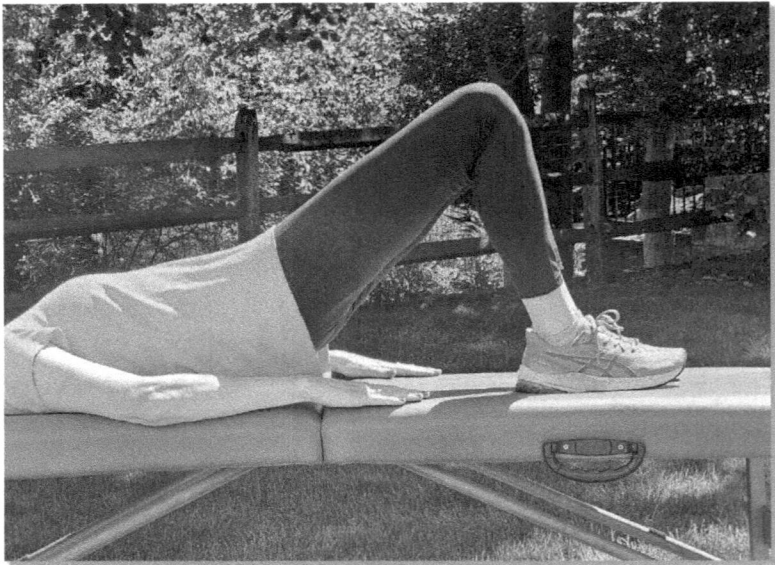

Figure 29 Bridging

Simple Back Stretches to Improve Lumbar Flexibility

Rocco groans. He went to bed feeling fine but woke up feeling tight and uncomfortable. After he walks around for five or ten minutes, the pain usually eases. He wonders if there are stretches he can do to increase the flexibility of the muscles and tissues in his lower back.

Muscles and soft tissues in the lumbar (low back) region can become tight, leading to pain, and limiting motion and mobility. Getting into a routine of gentle daily stretches can help decrease pain and increase your flexibility.

If you feel your back is tight or you want to increase your flexibility, aim to perform each of the stretches as noted. Make sure to relax briefly between each stretch. Don't bounce, as this may injure muscle fibers.

Pelvic tilt: Lie on your back with your knees bent and feet flat on the bed. Next, gently tighten your abdominal muscles (TrA) in the stomach area to rotate your pelvis to flatten your lower back. Imagine you have a glass of iced tea on your navel. Move your pelvis in a rocking motion to "spill" the iced tea toward your stomach. Hold for 5 seconds without holding your breath. Repeat 10 times, once per day.

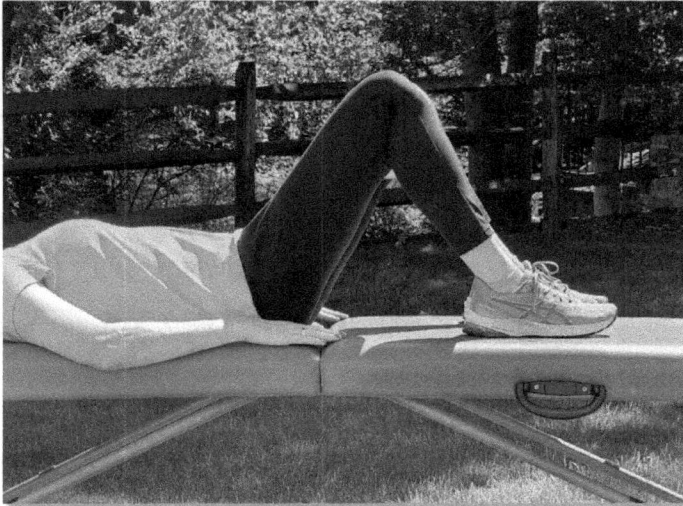

Figure 30 Pelvic tilt

Single knee-to-chest stretch: Lie on your back with your knees bent and your feet flat on the bed. Grab hold of one knee and gently pull it up toward your chest, while keeping the opposite knee in the bent position with the foot remaining flat on the bed. If you have trouble reaching your knees, you can use a towel to assist by placing the center of the towel at the back of your knee and using your hands to pull gently on the two towel ends. Hold for 5 seconds without holding your breath. Repeat 10 times, once per day.

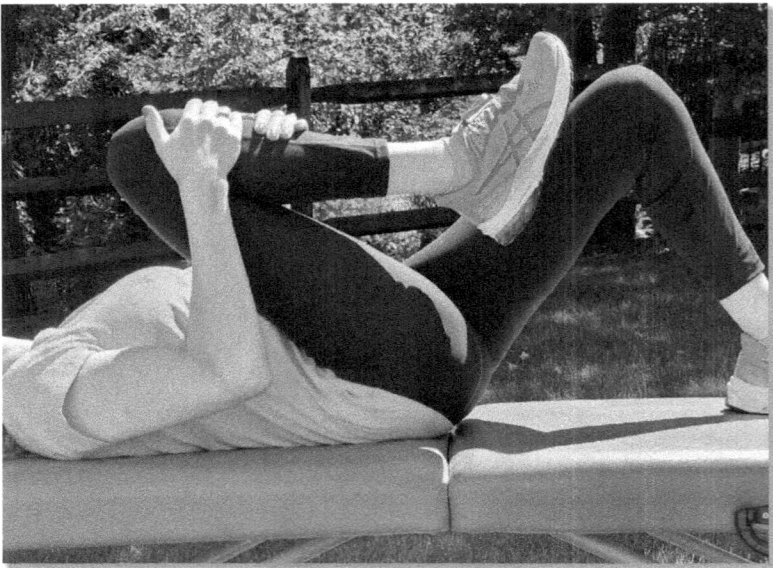

Figure 31 Single knee-to-chest stretch

Double knee-to-chest stretch: While lying on your back, hold both knees and gently pull them up toward your chest. You can also use a towel to assist you if necessary (as described in the single knee-to-chest stretch). Hold for 10 seconds without holding your breath. Repeat 10 times, once per day.

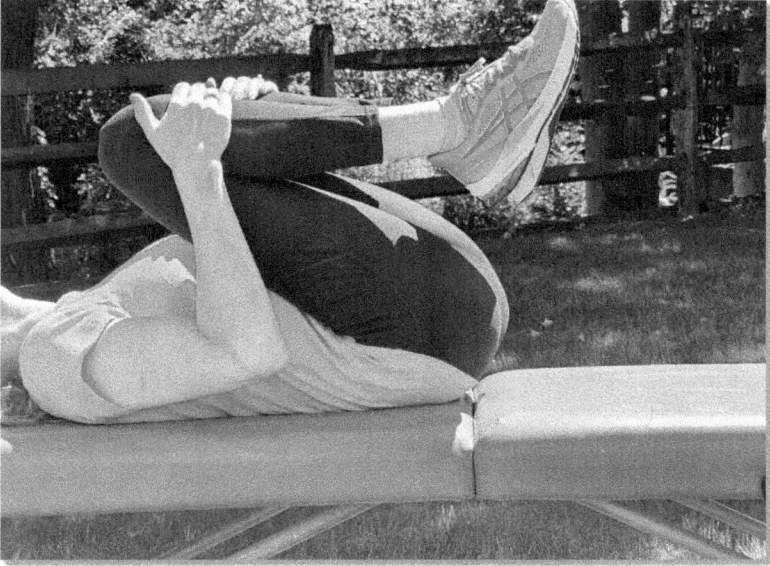

Figure 32 Double knee-to-chest stretch

Lower trunk rotation stretch: Lying on your back with your knees bent and your feet resting on the exercise mat, gently move both knees to one side until you feel a stretch. Hold 10 seconds and then move both knees to the other side until you feel a stretch in that direction. For an added stretch, turn your head in the opposite direction Of your knees. Continue to stretch each way for 10 repetitions with 10 second holds.

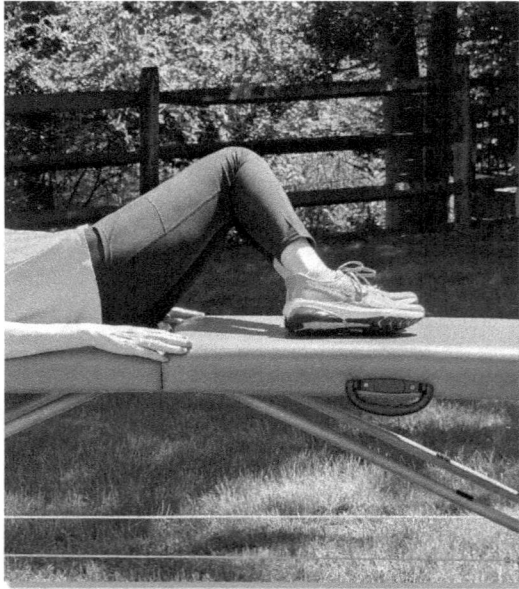

Figure 33 Lower trunk rotation stretch

Piriformis stretch: Your piriformis muscle is located in your buttock. While lying on your back, hold the outside of your right knee with your left hand and draw your knee up and over toward your left shoulder. Hold 30 seconds for 3 repetitions. Switch your hand position and repeat three times on the left leg.

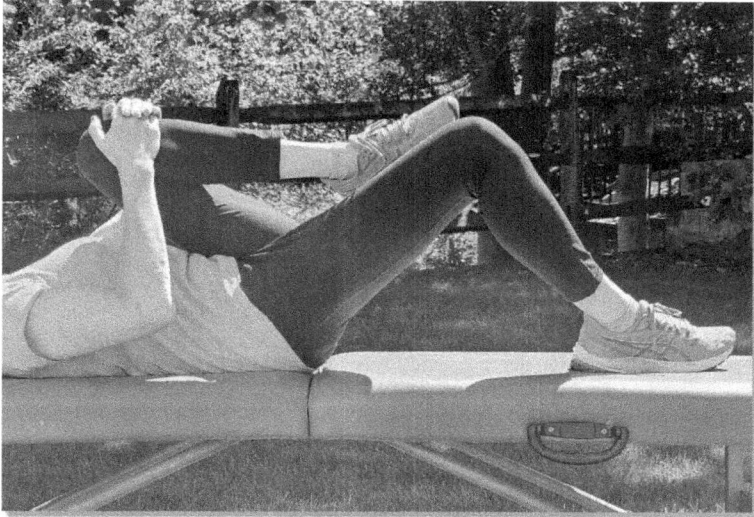

Figure 34 Piriformis stretch

Hamstring stretch: Your hamstrings muscles can be found on the back of your thigh. While lying down on your back, hook a towel or strap (a dog leash works well) under your foot. Keep your knee straight and draw up your leg until a stretch is felt in the back of your leg (hamstring/calf area). It's important to keep the opposite knee bent to limit stress in the lower back. Hold 30 seconds for 3 repetitions. If this position is uncomfortable for you, you can modify it by performing the stretch while standing. Place the leg you want to stretch on a footstool or bottom step of a staircase. Bend forward at your waist until you feel a stretch in the back of your thigh.

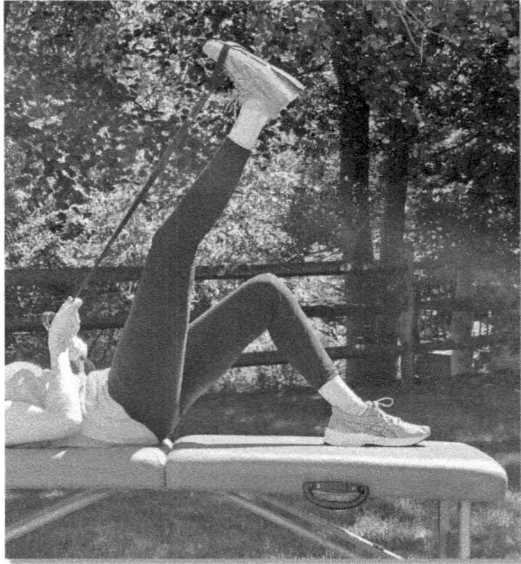

Figure 35 Hamstring stretch

Seeing Your Physician

If you have a sudden onset of pain in your lower back or pain which radiates into your buttocks or legs/feet, you should see your physician immediately. One red flag requiring an immediate visit to a doctor includes sudden weakness or numbness in one or both legs or feet. Another red flag is a sudden loss of bladder or bowel control. Your physician may need to rule out possible problems such as back-related tumors, infections, fractures, herniated discs, and Cauda Equina Syndrome (damage to the bundle of nerves below the end of the spinal cord). Mild, yet nagging back pain is also cause for a check-up.

Stretching and Strengthening the Neck and Upper Back

The average head weighs approximately 10-11 pounds. That's like having a bowling ball balanced on top of your shoulders. You need strong, flexible cervical (neck) muscles to be able to have good posture, lift objects, and turn and bend your neck. Muscle weakness and poor posture, such as a forward head and rounded shoulders, can lead to pain and impaired movement.

In general, there are three types of neck muscles: flexors, extensors, and oblique muscles. Flexors tend to be in the front of your neck. They allow you to bend your neck forward. Cervical extensors, which are in the back of your neck and upper back, allow you to stand up straight, lift, and reach. Oblique muscles, which are located on the sides of your neck, allow for rotation and side bending of the neck. All the muscles work together to enable proper posture. The muscles work with your ligaments to allow both movement (mobility) and stability.

The exercises below can help to keep your neck and upper back strong and flexible as you get older. They are not intended to cure pre-existing neck problems. If any of the exercises cause pain or worsen your existing pain, seek the advice of a physician or licensed physical therapist for guidance.

Cervical Strengthening Exercises

If you feel like your neck muscles are weak and that it is difficult for you to hold your head up, or if you feel fatigued when you try to maintain good posture, you can try performing the gentle isometric exercises described below. An isometric contraction is one in which you contract the involved muscles without moving the joints. In other words, as you perform the exercises below, your head will remain still. Hold each muscle contraction for 3 seconds and perform 8 to 10 repetitions of each exercise, once per day. Remember, don't hold your breath.

1. **Isometric Flexion:** Place the tips of your index and middle fingers on your forehead and gently push your head forward into your fingers. Your head should not move.
2. **Isometric Extension:** Place the tips of your index and middle fingers on the center of the back of your head and gently draw your head back into your fingers. Your head should not move.
3. **Isometric Side Bend:** Place the tips of your index and middle fingers on the side of your head and gently push your head into your fingers, as if you were trying to tilt it sideways. Your head should not move.
4. **Isometric Rotation:** Place the tips of your index and middle fingers on your cheek bone and gently push your head into your fingers, as if you were trying to rotate (turn) it. Your head should not move.

Have you ever been told that you have a forward head posture (FHP)? Good posture means that your ears are positioned over your shoulders. If you have poor posture, your head may shift forward over time. Exercises, such as the chin tuck described below, work to strengthen the deep cervical muscles located in the front of your neck. These muscles, which can become weak and easily fatigued in patients

144

with chronic neck pain, help to nod your head forward, turn, and bend. Chin tucks are a retraction exercise. That is, they help to move the head back over the shoulders. This type of exercise not only helps to strengthen the deep cervical muscles, but also to return them to their optimal length.

Chin Tuck: Start by sitting with an upright posture. Slowly draw your head back so that your ears line up with your shoulders, as if you are making yourself a "double chin." Do not nod your head. Hold for 3 seconds. Repeat 10 times, twice per day as tolerated. You can also perform this exercise while lying on your back with your knees bent (hook lying). If possible, do not use a pillow under your head and neck. Make sure to keep your mouth closed. Push the back of your head straight down into the floor or bed and hold for 3 seconds. Repeat 10 times, twice per day.

Seeing Your Physician

If you have a sudden onset of pain in your neck or pain which radiates into your shoulders or arms/hands, contact your physician immediately or call 911. Other red flags requiring an immediate visit to a doctor include a sudden weakness or numbness in one or both arms or hands. Your physician may need to rule out possible problems such as myocardial infarction (heart attack), instability of one or more ligaments of the neck region, spinal cord injury, or herniated disc, to name a few. Mild, yet nagging neck pain is also cause for a check-up.

Simple Stretches to Improve Neck and Upper Back Flexibility

Enrique Gomez dreads the day his children tell him he is too old to drive. He's always thought he might lose his driver's license if he becomes forgetful. Now, however, he realizes his neck is so stiff, he can't turn to look behind him when he's

145

backing up. If he doesn't figure out how to stretch his muscles and get better neck range of motion, he knows his driving days are numbered.

Just as with your low back, cervical (neck) and thoracic (upper back) muscles can become tight, leading to muscle spasms and pain. This limitation in muscle flexibility can make it difficult to perform everyday activities, such as turning your head while driving or trying to safely cross the road. Muscle tightness can lead to impaired blood circulation, which decreases nutrients to your muscles. As described previously, chronic poor posture can also lead to muscle tightness.

If you want to improve your neck range of motion and flexibility, try making the following exercises part of your daily routine.

1. **Cervical Rotation**: Rotate your head toward the side, then return back to looking straight ahead. Repeat to the opposite side. Hold 5 seconds and repeat 5-10 times, 1-2 times per day.

2. **Cervical Side Bend**: Tilt your head toward the side (bringing your head towards your shoulder), then return back to looking straight ahead. Repeat to the opposite side. Hold 5 seconds and repeat 5-10 times, 1-2 times per day.

3. **Cervical Extension**: Tilt your head upward, such that you are looking at the ceiling. Then return to looking straight ahead. If this exercise makes you dizzy, don't do it. Hold 5 seconds and repeat 5-10 times, 1-2 times per day.

4. **Cervical Flexion**: Tilt your head downward, such that you are looking at the floor. Then return to looking straight ahead. Hold 5 seconds and repeat 5-10 times, 1-2 times per day.

5. **Upper Trap Stretch**: Your trapezius muscles, which cover the back of your neck and upper back, include an upper, middle, and lower section. They move and rotate your shoulder blade, extend your neck, and stabilize your arm. Since they do so much work, they are susceptible to stress, strain, and excess tension. This is

particularly true for the upper traps. Begin by standing or sitting with good posture. To stretch the right traps, grab the bottom of your chair with your right hand. Then slowly tilt your head to the left side, bringing your left ear toward your left shoulder until you feel a gentle stretch along the right side of your neck and shoulder. Hold for 30 seconds. Repeat 3 times on each side.

6. **Scapular Retractions**: Start by sitting or standing with an upright posture. Squeeze your shoulder blades back and down toward your spine. Hold for 3 seconds and relax. Repeat 10 times.

7. **Levator Scapulae Stretch**: Begin by standing or sitting with good posture. To stretch your right levator scapulae, place your right hand on the top/back of your right shoulder to stabilize. Use your left hand to draw your head downward and toward the opposite side (in the direction of your armpit). Your left hand, which is assisting the stretch, should be placed on the back/top of your head. You should feel a stretch between the top of your right shoulder blade and behind your right ear. Hold for 30 seconds and repeat 3 times. Then, switch hand positions and perform 3 times in the opposite direction.

Thoracic (Middle Back) Stretches

Your upper back muscles also play a role in posture. These muscles may become tight, leading to pain or poor flexibility. Below are ways you can stretch them.

Cat and camel: While positioned on your hands and knees, raise your back and arch it toward the ceiling (like an angry cat). Next, return to a lowered position, letting your stomach sag towards the floor into a swayback position. Hold 5 seconds in each direction and repeat 10 times.

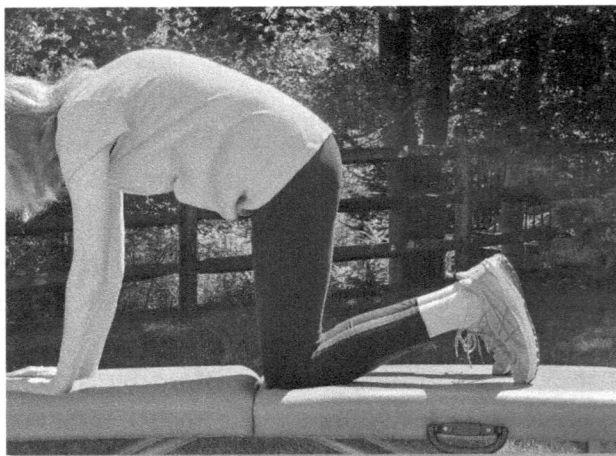

Figure 36 Cat and camel stretch (cat)

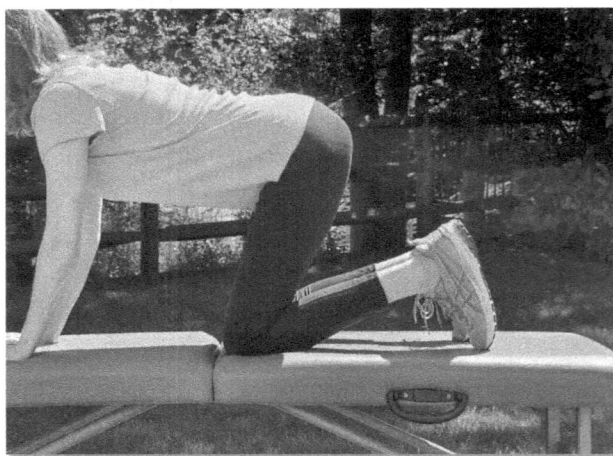

Figure 37 Cat and camel stretch (camel)

Prayer stretch: The prayer stretch targets the extensor muscles of the middle and low back. Since you'll be in a kneeling position for this stretch, you may wish to perform it on a padded surface or bed. Also, if you have knee problems or tightness, you can place a pillow between the backs of your thighs and calves while performing this stretch. To increase comfort, you can also let your feet hang over the edge of the bed. To begin, while on your hands and knees, slowly lower your buttocks toward your feet so that it is resting on your heels (or on the pillow) and slide your arms forward to lengthen your spine until a stretch is felt along your back. You can also slide your hands to either side (Lateral Prayer Stretch) to focus the stretch on the opposite side of your spine. Hold for 15 seconds and perform 3 repetitions. The prayer stretch needs to be approached with caution if you already have back pain. If you have severe knee pain, you may be unable to perform this stretch.

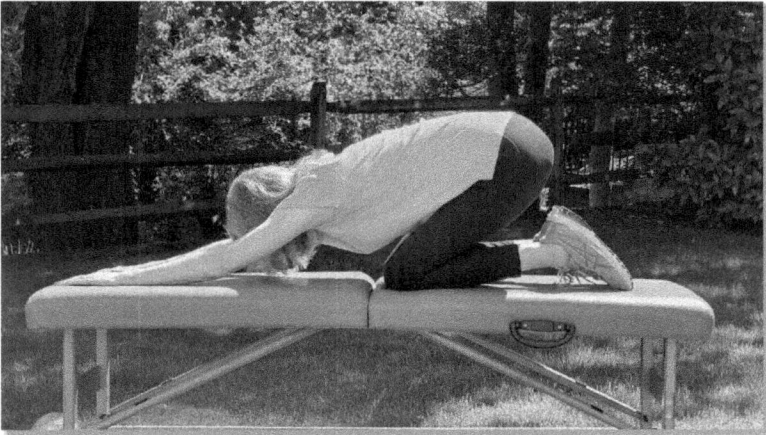

Figure 38 Prayer stretch

Seated upper trunk rotation: Cross your arms over your chest, then gently twist your trunk to one side. Hold 5 seconds and return to the starting position. Repeat 5-10 times in each direction.

Seated lateral trunk stretch: While in a seated position, raise your arm and reach over your head as you bend your trunk to the opposite side for a stretch. Hold 5 seconds and return to the starting position. Repeat 5-10 times in each direction.

Chapter 15

A Look at Osteoarthritis

*L*ila Martin's friends jokingly call her "the bionic woman." She has two new hips and two new knees. Her doctor recently mentioned replacing her left shoulder too. She is tired of surgery and isn't sure why all her joints seem to be giving out. She feels as though she is bringing the idea of "wear and tear" to a new level. Her new year's resolution is to make it through a whole year without having to get another joint replaced.

Osteoarthritis (OA) is the most common form of joint disease, sparing no age, race, or geographic area. At least 20 million adults in the United States suffer from the effects of this condition at any one time. About 90% of all people show evidence of OA on x-rays in weight-bearing joints such as the hips and knees by age 40.

OA doesn't happen overnight. It's characterized by degeneration (breaking down) of cartilage and by hypertrophy (building up) of bone at the articular margins. Articular cartilage is the tissue that covers the ends of bones where they come together to form a joint. As OA begins to develop, tiny areas of cartilage that cover the ends of bones soften and develop cracks or pitting. Eventually, larger pieces of cartilage wear away, leaving areas of bone bare. As the articular cartilage is worn away, the bones may begin grinding together. Loss of cartilage can cause the joint to lose its normal shape. The bone ends thicken, and bone spurs form along the joint margins. Cysts may form in the bone near the joint. As OA progresses, bone or cartilage fragments may float in the joint space. Inflammation may be present, especially with acute involvement of the finger joints.

Signs and Symptoms of Osteoarthritis

Do you feel pain or stiffness first thing in the morning or after resting? These are two common symptoms of OA. Pain can range from aching to a sharp or burning sensation. It is often worse after prolonged activity or towards the end of the day. Sometimes, arthritic pain can interfere with sleep. A sign of arthritic joints includes mild swelling. Range of motion may be limited, though stiffness may go away with activity. Joints may even become deformed. The muscles around an arthritic joint may grow weak, especially surrounding the knees. It's not uncommon to hear clicking, crunching, creaking, or cracking sounds when an arthritic joint bends. Symptoms usually build up gradually over time, rather than occurring suddenly.

Pain, swelling, and stiffness related to OA can make it challenging to perform normal activities of daily living at home. They can interfere with your ability to perform your job. Arthritis of the hip, knee or foot can make walking and stair climbing difficult. Arthritis of the hands can make it difficult to prepare meals, clean the house, type, write, sew/knit, etc. Neck and back arthritis can impact driving, reaching, and lifting.

Recall that spinal nerves branch off from the spinal cord. These spinal nerves pass through bony openings on the sides of the spine. Arthritis may narrow these openings, leading to a condition known as spinal stenosis. Spinal stenosis can cause pressure on the spinal cord or spinal nerves, leading to pain, weakness, and/or numbness.

Hip and Knee Arthritis

OA is the most common disorder affecting the hip and is also commonly seen at the knee joint. Primary OA is due to aging, while secondary OA is caused by disease or trauma (like a fall or car accident). Although one might think OA forms from too much stress through the joint, it can also form from not having enough weight-bearing through the hips and knees. Intermittent compression is needed to maintain healthy cartilage. When there are less compressive forces through the hip or knee joint because a person is less active and not bearing as much weight on their legs as they used to, cartilage begins to break down.

Older people may move around less and in smaller ranges of motion in their daily activities. This may cause some parts of the articular cartilage to not be subjected to normal stresses. Unfortunately, this predisposes them to developing OA. Degenerative changes can also be due to leg length discrepancy, tightness of the joint capsule, and obesity.

Specifically, people with OA of the hips often feel pain in the groin area or buttocks and sometimes on the inside of the knee or thigh. Those with OA of the knees may feel a grating, scraping, or grinding sensation when moving the knee. Preserving and building muscle mass may aid people in preserving walking and mobility.

Protecting Your Joints

Nowadays, it seems like getting total hip and total knee replacements is almost an epidemic. What can you do to protect your joints and try to reduce the odds that you'll get OA and require a joint replacement in the future?

First, modify your environment to avoid repetitive movements, such as bending. When certain motions are repeated several times a day over the course of months and years, the combined effect can harm your joints. These repetitive strain injuries can contribute to the eventual development of arthritis. You can also change your environment by using assistive devices, such as a raised toilet seat, a shower chair, or a long-handled reacher.

Next, avoid further wear and tear of your joints. Utilize good body mechanics in your daily activities. Use the largest, most stable joints possible for a task. This means lifting with your hips and knees, rather than using your back muscles. It's easier to push an item like a shopping cart than to pull it. Wear comfortable shoes with low heels which support and cushion your arches. Carpets can aid in cushioning the forces on your joints. Just make sure they are tacked down or slip-resistant for safety.

Vary your joint position frequently. If you must sit for a prolonged period of time, such as at a movie or a long car ride, occasionally move your joints by marching in your seat, kicking your legs, and wiggling your feet. Sit with your knees and hips in a relaxed position. If you have to stand for a prolonged period of time, you can intermittently shift your weight from side to side to rest the joints.

If an activity results in persistent pain, it's best to avoid it. If you notice fatigue, stop, and take a rest. Rest can significantly improve how you and your joints feel. Aim for eight to nine hours of sleep each night. It's helpful to use a pillow between your knees when lying on your side. While sleeping, try to keep your joints in good alignment to prevent tightening and loss of range of motion.

Hot and cold packs can help decrease pain and soreness. In addition, hot packs can reduce stiffness, and cold packs may lessen inflammation. Limit use to 20 minutes at a time for maximal benefits and to avoid injury (burns from hot packs or frostbite from cold packs). Take special care when using hot or cold packs if you have impaired sensation (for example, if you have diabetic neuropathy).

Organizing your tasks by planning ahead saves time and energy. Schedule your activities across the week rather than bunching them together on the same days. In other words, pace yourself. When grocery shopping, bring a list to stay organized and avoid unnecessary walking.

It's of vital importance to exercise safely. Proper exercise can strengthen the surrounding musculature or improve flexibility and therefore place less stress on the joints. Before beginning an exercise program, check with your physician for approval. Low impact exercises, such as walking or swimming are the safest way to start a program. For the best results, exercise regularly. If you have questions or concerns, you can obtain the advice of a personal trainer. If you already have signs or symptoms of OA, it may be best to seek the guidance of a physical therapist.

Exercises to Strengthen and Stretch the Hip and Knee

Is it an effort to climb stairs? Is it becoming difficult to keep up with your grandchildren or pets? Are you trying to regain your strength after an illness? Perhaps you are dreaming of taking up rock climbing. Regardless of your goals, keeping your legs strong and flexible is an important part of staying healthy as your hair starts turning silver. Following are some simple exercises to improve strength and flexibility.

Hip and Knee Strengthening Exercises

3-Way Straight Leg Raise: This is actually three exercises in one (straight leg raise, hip abduction, and hip extension). You can perform the exercises lying down or standing up. Perform 2 sets of 10 repetitions on each leg, 2 to 3 times per week. Please refer to the following photographs and descriptions for further details.
*Note: To increase the difficulty of the exercises, you may add cuff weights around your ankles. Gradually increase the weight as tolerated.

Supine (Lying Down):

Straight leg raise: While lying on your back with one knee bent, raise your other leg with a straight knee about 10-12 inches off the surface. Slowly lower.

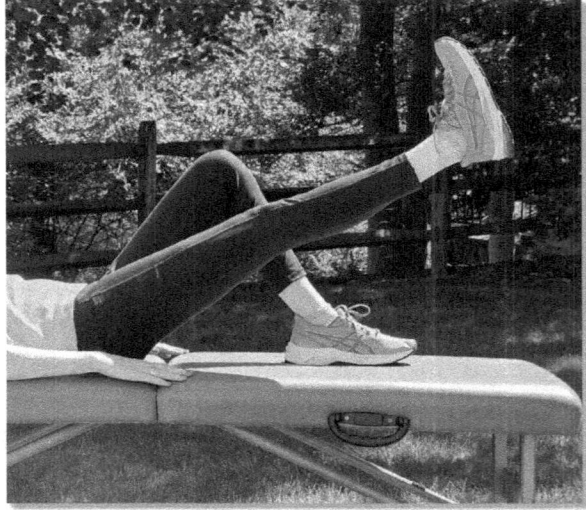

Figure 39 Straight leg raise

Hip abduction: While lying on your side, slowly raise your top leg up toward the ceiling. Keep your knee straight and keep your kneecap and toes pointed forward. You may keep your bottom leg bent to stabilize yourself. When you have completed 2 sets of 10 repetitions, turn to your other side and repeat with the other leg.

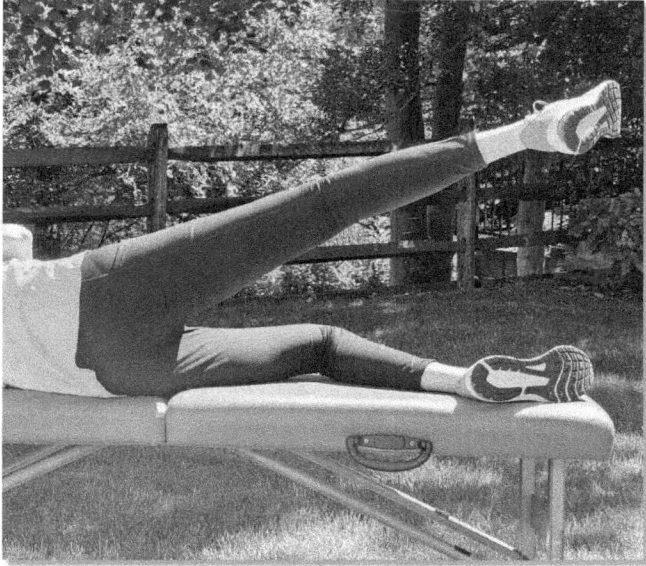

Figure 40 Hip abduction

Prone hip extension: While lying face down with your knee straight, slowly raise up your leg toward the ceiling and off the surface. Do not rotate or move your low back.

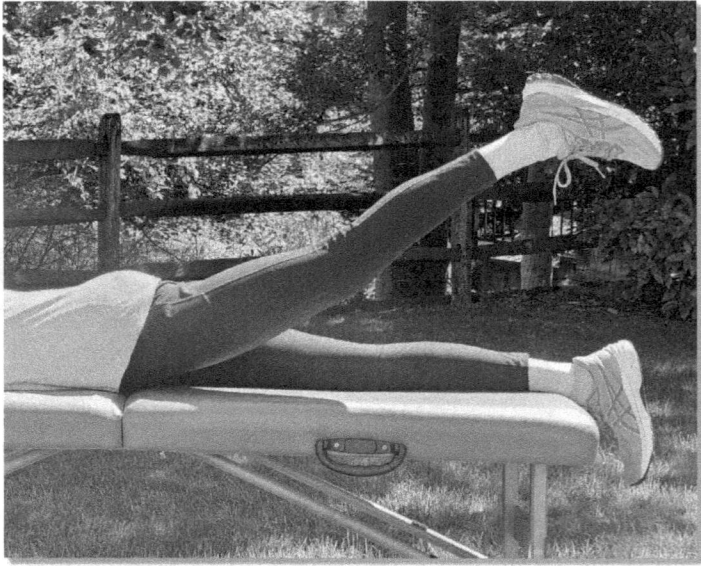

Figure 41 Prone hip extension

Standing Up: If you choose to perform the 3-Way Straight Leg Raise standing, you can hold onto a counter or sturdy high back chair for balance. Aim to perform 2 sets of 10 repetitions, 2 to 3 times per week. Add cuff weights around your ankles as tolerated. Start with a low weight and build up gradually to avoid strain or injury.

Straight leg raise: While standing, raise your leg forward, bending your hip about 45 degrees.

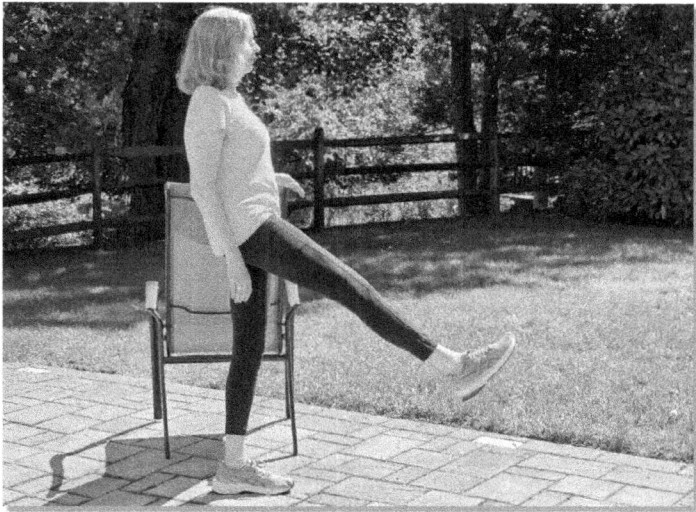

Figure 42 Standing straight leg raise

Hip abduction: While standing, raise your leg out to the side. Keep your knee straight and maintain your toes pointed forward. *Please refer to Figure 18.*

Hip extension: While standing, move your leg back while keeping your knee straight. Make sure to move only at your hip, and don't bend your trunk forward. *Please refer to Figure 19.*

Additional Supine (Lying Down) Hip and Knee Strengthening Exercises: Aim to perform each exercise 2 sets of 10 repetitions, 2 to 3 times per week.

Short arc quad: Place a rolled towel or small bolster under your knees. Slowly straighten your knee and raise your foot from the surface. Repeat on the other leg.

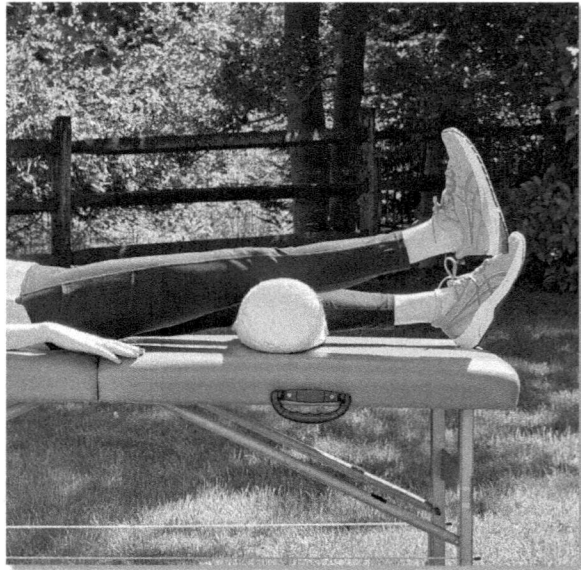

Figure 43 Short arc quad

Bridging: Lie on your back with your knees bent and your feet flat on the bed/mat. Pull in your navel like you are zipping up a tight pair of pants, then tighten your buttock muscles and raise your buttocks off the floor/bed (creating a "bridge" with your body). Hold for 3 seconds, relax, and repeat. *Please refer to Figure 29.*

Ball squeeze: Lie on your back with your knees bent and your feet flat on the surface. Place a small pillow, ball, or rolled up towel between your knees. Pull in your navel like you are zipping up a tight pair of pants and squeeze the object firmly between your knees. Hold for 3 seconds, relax, and repeat.

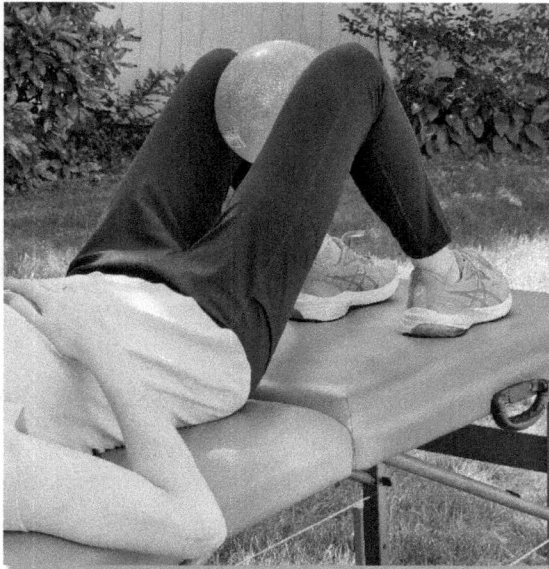

Figure 444 Ball squeeze

Clamshell with elastic band: Lie on your back with your knees bent and your feet flat on the surface. Place an elastic exercise band around your legs, just above the knees. Pull in your navel like you are zipping up a tight pair of pants and draw your knees apart against the resistance of the band. Slowly return and repeat.

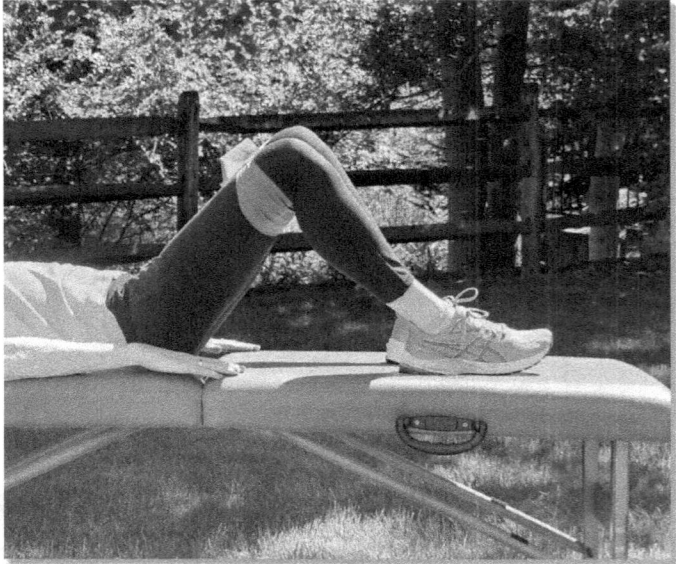

Figure 455 Clamshell with elastic band

Additional Standing Hip and Knee Strengthening Exercises: Use your arms for balance by holding a counter or high back chair as needed. Repeat each exercise 2 sets of 10 repetitions (unless otherwise noted), 2 to 3 times per week.

Heel raise: While standing, raise up on your toes as you lift your heels off the ground. Then, slowly lower your heels back down. Use a stable surface for support if needed. Start with 10 repetitions on each leg and build up to 20. *Please refer to Figure 21.*

Mini squat: While standing with your feet shoulder width apart (holding a counter or chair if needed), bend your knees and lower your body towards the floor. Your weight should mainly be directed through the heels of your feet. When bending, your knees should not go past your toes. Instead, pretend you are sitting in a chair and bring your buttocks backward. Return to standing position. Start with 10 repetitions on each leg and build up to 20. *Please refer to Figure 20.*

Hamstring curl: While standing, bend your knee so that your heel moves toward your buttock. Add cuff weights around your ankles as tolerated.

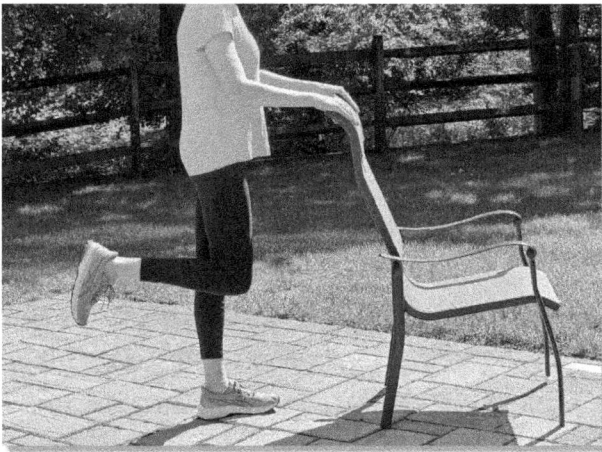

Figure 466 Hamstring curl

Step-up: You can use the bottom step of a staircase for this exercise. Hold the railing(s) for support/balance. Step up one step with your right leg and then with your left, such that both feet are on the step. Then step down with your left leg, followed by the right. Repeat 10 times and then switch legs, stepping up first with the left leg and down with the right. Make sure to use your leg muscles and avoid pulling yourself up with your arm muscles. Start with 10 repetitions on each leg and build up to 20.

Hip and Knee Stretches to Increase Flexibility

If you wish to increase hip and knee flexibility, try performing the following stretches on most days of the week.

Hamstring stretch: Your hamstrings muscles can be found on the back of your thigh. While lying down on your back, hook a towel or strap (like a dog leash) under your foot. Keep your knee straight and draw up your leg until a stretch is felt in the back of your leg (hamstring/calf area). It is important to keep the opposite knee bent to limit stress in the lower back. Hold 30 seconds for 3 repetitions on each leg.

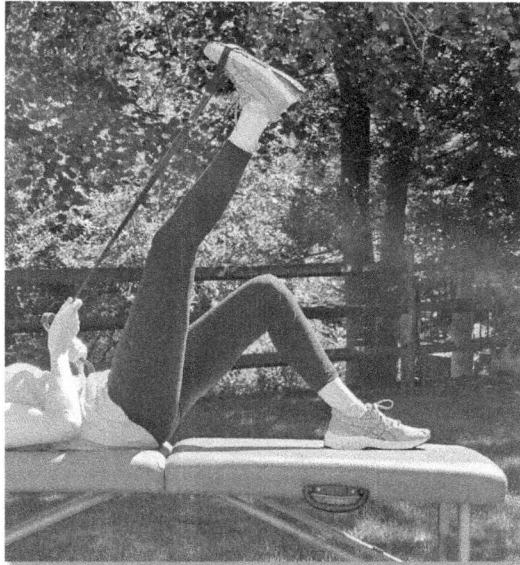

Figure 47 Hamstring stretch

Piriformis stretch: The piriformis muscle, which helps to rotate the hip outwards, is located in the buttock. A tight piriformis muscle can compress the sciatic nerve, causing pain in the buttock which may radiate down the leg. To stretch this muscle, lie on your back with your knees bent and your feet flat on the surface. To stretch your right piriformis, hold the outside of your right knee with your left hand, and draw your right knee up and over toward your left shoulder. Hold 30 seconds for 3 repetitions on each side. *Please refer to Figure 34.*

Quadriceps stretch: Your quadriceps muscles are on the front of your thighs. Hold onto a counter or sturdy chair with your left hand (for balance). Then, standing on your left leg, raise the right foot behind you, bending the knee. Use your right hand to pull the right foot as close to your buttocks as possible. If you cannot reach your foot, you can use a belt or strap to help you. Alternatively, this stretch can be performed in a sidelying position. Hold 30 seconds for 3 repetitions on each side.

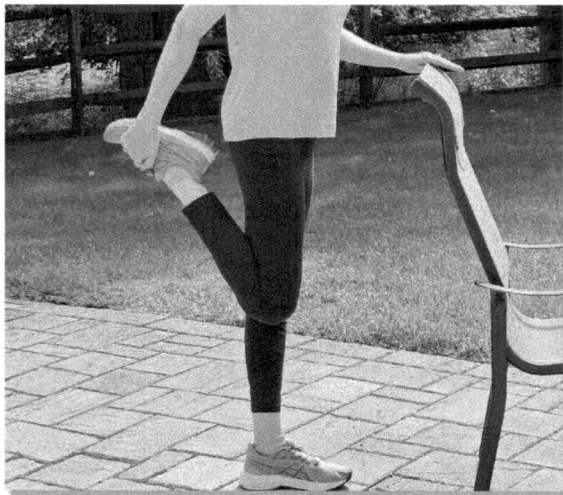

Figure 48 Quadriceps stretch

Butterfly stretch: This stretches the adductor muscles, which are located on the inside of your thighs. Lie on your back with your knees bent and feet together (flat on the surface). Lower your knees to the sides to stretch your inner thighs. Don't hold your breath while you stretch. Hold 30 seconds for 3 repetitions.

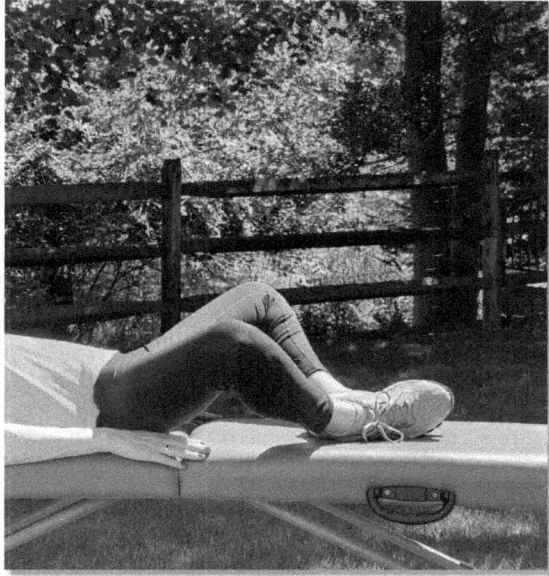

Figure 49 Butterfly stretch

Calf stretch with a towel or strap: Your calf muscles include your gastrocnemius and soleus muscles, which are located on the back of your lower leg. While in a seated position, hook a towel, strap, or dog leash under your foot and pull your ankle back until you feel a stretch in your calf area. Keep your knee straight during the stretch. Don't hold your breath while stretching. Hold 30 seconds for 3 repetitions on each side.

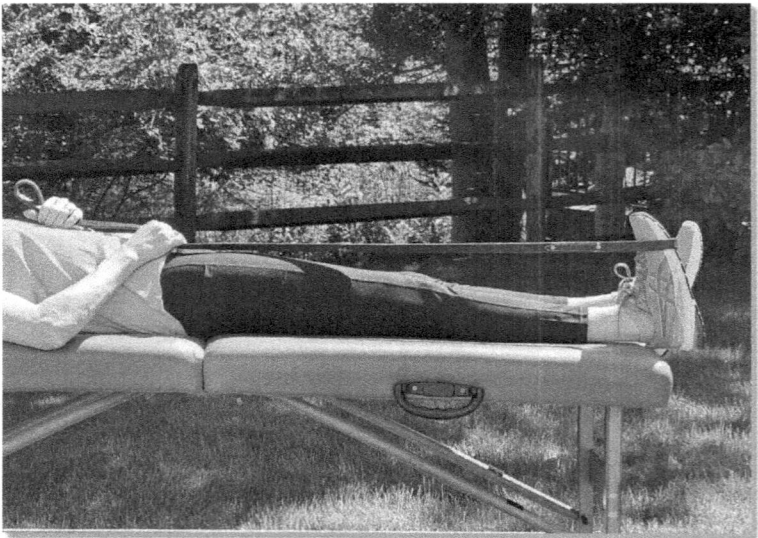

Figure 470 Calf stretch with towel or strap

ITB (Ilio-Tibial Band): The ITB is a thick band of fibrous tissue that runs down the outside of your leg from the iliac crest of your pelvis, the tensor fascia lata muscle, and the gluteal (buttock) muscles to your knee. Tightness of the ITB can make subtle changes in the way the knee moves, resulting in pain. Tightness may also cause maltracking (improper gliding) of the patella (kneecap). It can also irritate the bursa, which are small fluid filled sacs that provide cushioning between the ITB and the bones below. The stretch: Hold onto a chair or counter as needed for balance. Stand upright and cross your right leg behind your left. Next, with your arms overhead, lean towards the left until you feel the ITB stretch on the outside of your right leg. Hold for 30 seconds for 3 repetitions on each side.

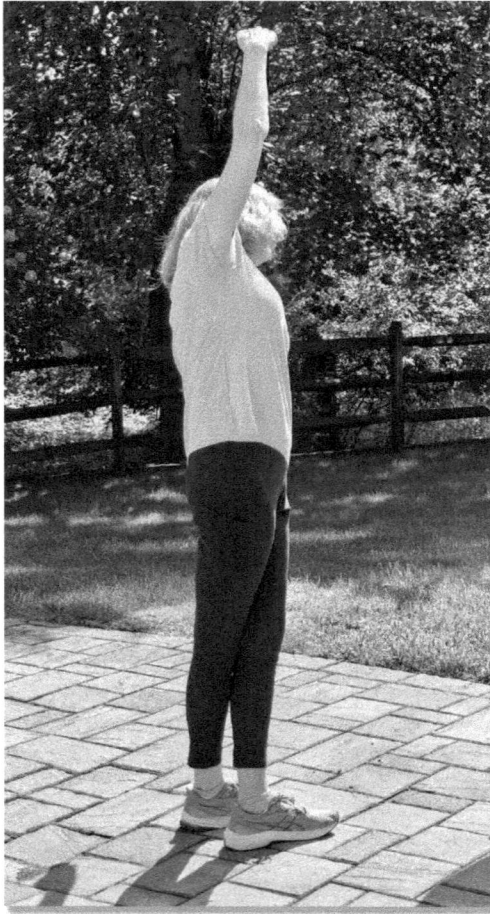

Figure 481 Ilio-tibial (ITB) stretch

Getting a Grip on Hand Pain and Stiffness

Eliza loves knitting. Currently, she is working on a baby blanket for her third grandchild. However, she is having trouble finishing it due to pain and stiffness in her fingers. It is also growing difficult to type emails to her friends. Should she try putting ice or a heating pad on her hands? Would aspirin or ibuprofen help? Perhaps it is time to call her physician.

Have you noticed bumps form on your finger joints? Have your fingers started to become "crooked?" When you wake up, do your hands feel stiff? If yes, you may have osteoarthritis of the hands. This can make it difficult to perform activities such as house cleaning, cooking, working on your computer, writing, sewing, and knitting. Bony growths (spurs) at the edge of joints can cause fingers to become swollen, tender and red. If the bumps are on the joint closest to the fingernail, they are called Heberden's nodes. If they are near the middle joint of the finger, they are referred to as Bouchard's nodes. Another common site for arthritic hand pain is at the base of the thumb.

Do you have pain, numbness, or tingling in your wrist or hand? This can be a sign of carpal tunnel syndrome (CTS), a common overuse injury involving compression on the median nerve at the wrist. It can make it difficult to perform activities of daily living, like buttoning your shirt or holding a cup. A "tunnel" is formed on the underside of your wrist by non-elastic bands of tissue and your wrist (carpal) bones. If pressure is placed on the nerve due to swelling inside the tunnel from osteoarthritis, tendon inflammation (tendonitis), pain, and numbness may result.

CTS is a repetitive stress syndrome. To prevent it or lessen the symptoms, try to avoid activities which stress the wrist, such as tight gripping, pinching, repeated bending of the wrist up and down, and holding the wrist in a flexed (downward bent) position. Organize your office and work areas to maximize proper posture and decrease stress on your neck, shoulders, and wrists. Support your forearms when doing work involving your hands. For example, use an ergonomic wrist pad and mouse pad when typing. If you have significant symptoms, your physician or therapist may prescribe a resting wrist splint.

Modify Your Activities to Decrease
Hand Pain and Fatigue

In general, it's helpful to avoid positions that foster deformity of the fingers and hands. What does this mean? Activities such as tight pinching, tight gripping, excessive or constant pressure on the joints, and prolonged static hand postures can worsen hand pain and arthritis.

What are some simple ways to lessen joint strain? When possible, pick up a mug using two hands rather than gripping the handle tightly between your thumb and fingers of one hand. If you can, pick up objects between your palms rather than with curled fingers. Avoid resting your chin on your knuckles, since this position increases strain. Carry your purse over your shoulder or forearm, rather than carrying it with your hand.

In the kitchen, put frequently used items on easy to reach shelves. Use small, lightweight containers instead of heavy, bulky ones. When possible, choose lightweight utensils over heavy skillets. Electric appliances, such as can openers, are easier on your hands than manual ones. If necessary, use foot operated devices, such as garbage cans, to decrease use of your hands. Long lever arms on faucets are easier to use than small knobs. Likewise, you can build up the handles on cooking utensils using Dycem to make them larger and softer. This allows you to exert less effort.

When washing counters, use a flat hand and avoid gripping the sponge or cleaning cloth tightly. To remove excess water from a sponge or cloth, push it with a flat hand against the sink surface rather than wringing it out. If you have trouble opening jars, try using a flat hand and turning the lid toward your thumb side of your hand. If this technique isn't enough, there are tools available (adaptive equipment) designed to help you. Are you a cook, but hand pain is holding you back? You may benefit from a cutting board with special prongs in it that stabilize fruits and vegetables, making it easier to cut them.

If you're like most people, you don't get excited about house cleaning. Housekeeping can put strain on your hands. Divide chores across the days of the week. Encourage family members to help. It helps to purchase lightweight equipment for cleaning. A sponge mop is easier to squeeze out than one that requires wringing. A laundry cart with wheels makes it easier to get clothing and bedding to and from the washer and dryer.

What about yard work? When sweeping or raking, keep your back straight and the handle out in front of you. Keep your knuckles parallel to the handle. Make sure your hands are holding the handle above waist level in order to avoid poor posture and strain.

Getting dressed can be difficult for people with hand pain or weakness. Clothing with front openings with zippers or large buttons may be helpful. A buttonholer is an inexpensive tool that's used to manage buttons. Likewise, zipper pulls can be added to small, difficult to grasp zippers. Mittens are easier to don than gloves. If one arm is weaker or more painful than the other, dress that side first (e.g., the painful arm goes into the coat sleeve first). If you need to wear a belt, loop it through the pants before you don them. Women can opt to choose bras with front closures. If needed, purchase elastic laces for shoes.

Adaptive equipment can also help relieve some of the strain on arthritic hands. For example, keys can be built up to create a larger handle. This creates a longer lever arm and allows you to rotate your arm to turn the key, rather than using just your fingers. A foam steering wheel cover makes the wheel larger and softer, thus enabling you to use a less forceful grip.

If you have questions or concerns regarding hand pain or related symptoms, contact your health care provider, an occupational therapist, or a physical therapist for an examination and medical advice. Keep reading for some simple hand range of motion and strengthening exercises.

Simple Exercises for Hand Range of Motion

If you suffer from osteoarthritis of the hand, there are a few simple active range of motion (AROM) exercises you can perform each day. These should help ease pain and stiffness as well as increase blood flow to the hands. Aim to perform each exercise 10 times, 1-2 times per day.

Towel scrunches: Place your hand palm down on a hand or dish towel. Maintaining contact between the heel of your hand and the surface of the towel, scrunch the towel by bending your fingers.

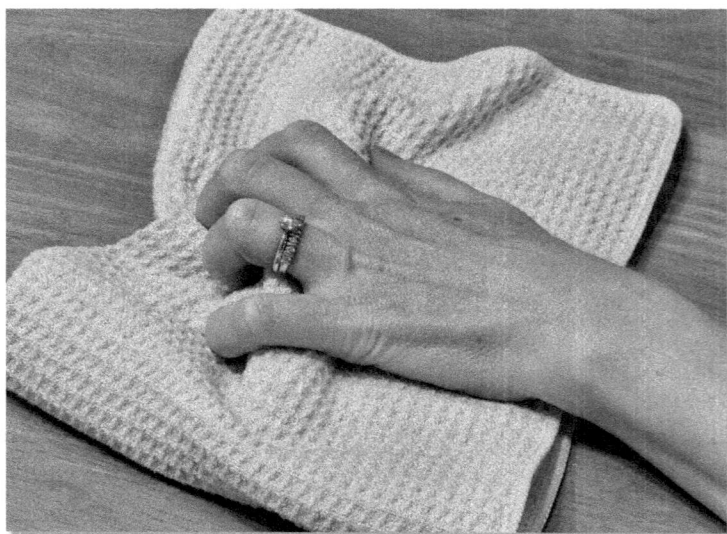

Figure 51 Towel scrunches

Finger spread: With your hand flat on a table, spread your fingers apart, then bring them together as close as possible.

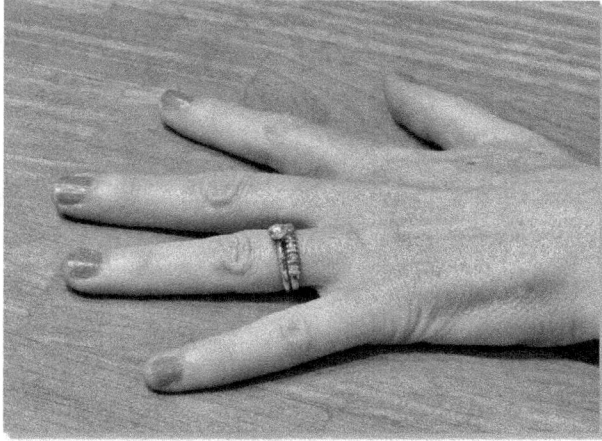

Figure 492 Finger spread

Finger raises: With your palm on a table, straighten your fingers completely at the large knuckles and lift your fingers off the table.

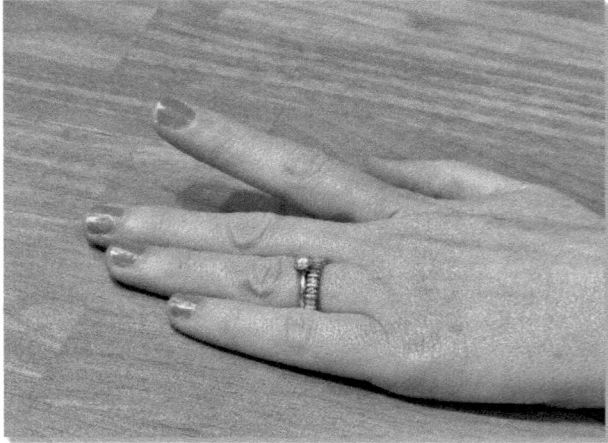

Figure 53 Finger raises

Hand/Wrist Stretches

Hold each of the following stretches for 5 seconds and repeat 5 times, once per day. Be gentle!

Active wrist flexor stretch: Hold your arm such that your palm is facing away from you. Keep your elbow straight. Using your other hand, gently bend your wrist upwards.

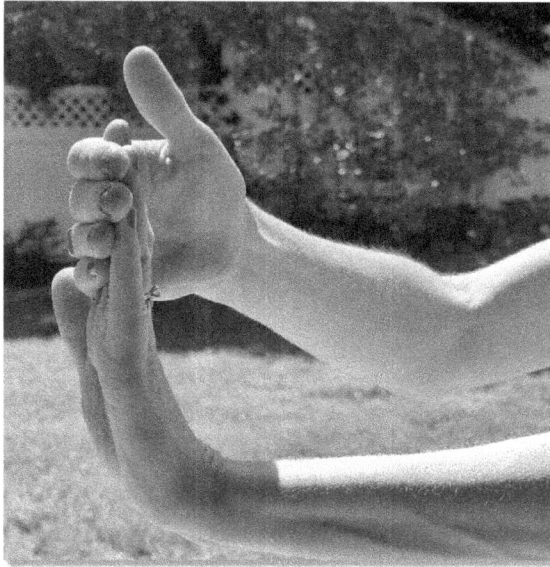

Figure 54 Active wrist flexor stretch

Active wrist extensor stretch: Hold your arm such that your palm is facing downward. Keep your elbow straight. Using your other hand, gently bend your wrist downwards.

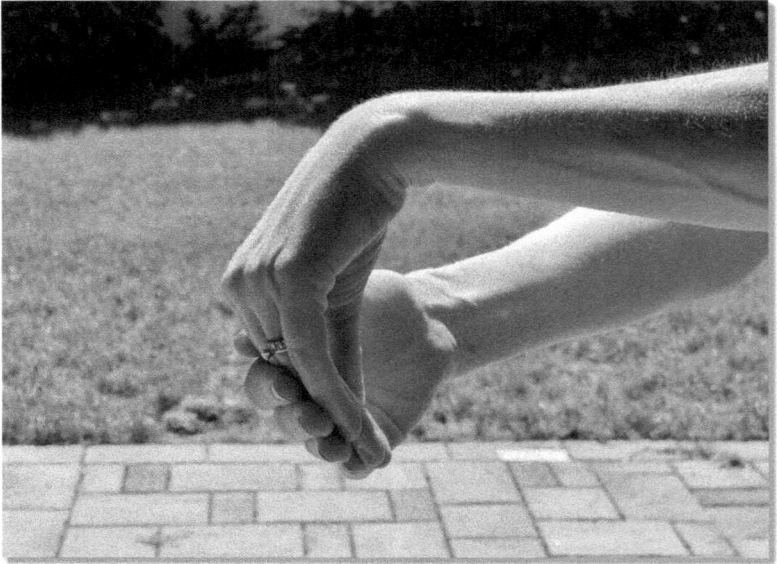

Figure 55 Active wrist extensor stretch

Finger stretch: Bend only your fingertips until they touch the upper part of your palm. Keep your large knuckles straight.

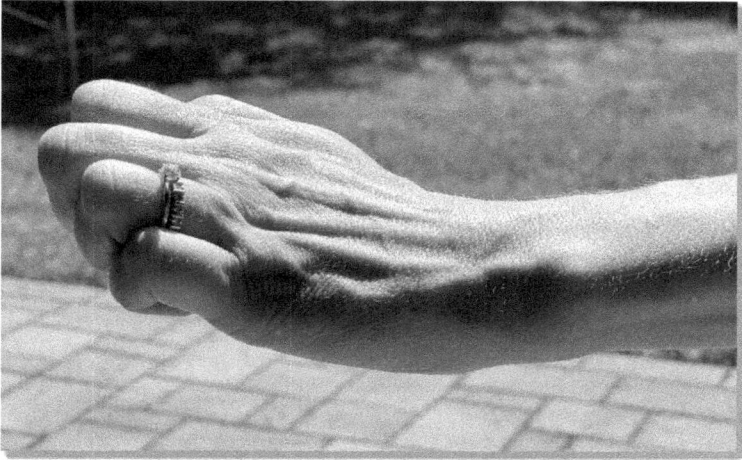

Figure 56 Finger stretch

Hand Strengthening Exercises

The following exercises are designed to strengthen the muscles of your hands. Hold each squeeze for 3 seconds. Perform 3 times per week. Avoid over-fatiguing the muscles. If your hands are painful or arthritic, the range of motion exercises above may be more beneficial than strengthening. If you are unsure, consult with your physician, physical therapist, or occupational therapist.

1. **Putty Squeeze**: Squeeze resistive putty for 3 seconds. Repeat 10 times.
2. **Putty Roll**: Roll the resistive putty back and forth on a table, making sure all your fingertips are used. Roll the putty for 5 seconds and repeat 10 times.
3. **Table Squeeze**: Squeeze the edge of a table between your fingers and your thumb for 3 seconds. Your fingers should

be on top of the table, and your thumb should be on the bottom of the table. Keep your fingers bent only at the large knuckles. Repeat 10 times.

Part IV: Healthy Aging from the Outside In

Chapter 16

Avoiding Skin Cancer and Keeping Your Youthful Appearance

*R*andy picks at the scab at his hairline. It oozes a bit of fluid, so he dabs it with *a tissue. It started as a small red spot four months ago, which at the time, he thought was a pimple. The crusty scab came and went. He's gotten a few severe sunburns over the years. He decides it is time to see a dermatologist for a full-body exam for skin cancer.*

Think you can't get skin cancer? Think again. Twenty percent of Americans will develop it by the time they reach the age of seventy.[1] More than 58 million Americans have actinic keratosis, a common precursor to skin cancer marked by dry, scaly spots or patches.[2] Knowing the signs and symptoms of skin cancer can help you recognize it sooner. That way, it's easier to treat.

What is skin cancer? In a nutshell, it's the abnormal growth of skin cells. Although people who have light skin have a higher risk, people of all colors and races can develop skin cancer. Basal cell carcinoma (BCC) is the most common type of skin cancer. It often appears as a small flesh-colored shiny bump, but it can also be open sores or pink/red patches. Although they rarely spread, they should be treated promptly.

Squamous cell carcinoma (SCC), the second most common type of skin cancer, may present as a scaly patch of skin, a firm red bump, a wart, or a non-healing sore which may ooze or bleed. If not treated promptly, it can spread and become life-threatening.

Both BCC and SCC are most commonly found on parts of the body that receive a lot of sun exposure (e.g., face/head, arms/hands, and neck), but they can be found anywhere on the body. They are more common in lighter skinned individuals, but they can appear in darker skinned people as well. When caught early enough, both types are highly treatable.

Melanoma is the deadliest kind of skin cancer. In fact, one person dies from it every hour.[3] Like basal cell and squamous cell carcinoma, it's most often due to sun exposure. If you've had more than five sunburns, your risk of melanoma doubles.[4] If you want to read more frightening statistics, visit www.skincancer.org.[5]

Melanoma can develop within a mole, but more often occurs as a dark spot on previously healthy skin. It's the skin cancer that's most likely to spread to other organs. Survival rates are higher with early diagnosis and treatment, so quick intervention is crucial.

The website of the American Academy of Dermatologists (www.aad.org) includes detailed instructions for examining your skin for cancer.[6] They suggest studying your skin in front of a large mirror, with the assistance of an additional hand-held mirror. Dermatologists developed the concept of ABCDE to aid in screening for melanoma.

Asymmetry: If you draw an imaginary line through the center, one half is different from the other half. In other words, one part of the mole or suspicious skin lesion doesn't match the rest.

Border: Melanoma has irregular or poorly defined edges or borders that may be ragged or blurred.

Color: The colors within a melanoma can vary and may range from beige/brown or black to white, pink/red, or even blue.

Diameter: The classic reference for the size of a melanoma is that the diameter is often larger than a standard pencil eraser (6mm or ¼ inch), but they can be smaller.

Evolving: The area may be growing or changing in color, shape, or size. If it's a mole, it may look different from the other ones you have.

Take advantage of free skin cancer screenings in your community. If you have any questions or concerns, ask your doctor, or visit a dermatologist. For example, point out any new spots, changes in pre-existing moles, or moles that don't appear like others on your body. Notify your doctor of non-healing sores. Be sure to mention areas that are itchy, painful, or tender or that have oozing, bleeding, or scales.

The majority of skin cancers are due to the sun. In addition, 90% of skin aging is caused by the sun. In my years as a physical therapist, I've had numerous patients mention they got skin cancer on the left side of their face, their left neck, and left arm from many hours spent driving, often for work. Remember, the harmful rays of the sun can penetrate car windows. UV radiation from the sun includes UVA and UVB rays. It reaches earth as long wavelength ultraviolet A (UVA) and shortwave ultraviolet B (UVB) rays. Glass blocks UVB, and windshields are specially treated to block UVA. However, UVA rays can penetrate a car's side and rear windows.

It's never too late to limit your exposure. The Skin Cancer Foundation, formed in 1979, is an excellent resource for tips about protection from the sun.[5] Their skin cancer prevention tips include:

- Seek the shade, especially between 10 AM and 4 PM. This is when the sun's rays are at their strongest. If you're at the beach, pool, or a sunny sporting event, take breaks from the sun whenever possible.
- Avoid sunburns.
- Steer clear from tanning and UV tanning beds. More people develop skin cancer from indoor tanning than lung cancer from smoking.[7] Even occasional tanning bed use triples the risk of skin cancer.
- Cover up with clothing, including a broad-brimmed hat and UV-blocking sunglasses.
- Use a broad spectrum (UVA/UVB) sunscreen with an SPF of 15 or higher every day. It's important to block both UVA and UVB rays since both can be harmful.

- For longer outdoor activities, choose a water-resistant, broad spectrum (UVA/UVB) sunscreen with an SPF of 30 or higher. Make sure it hasn't gone past the expiration date.
- Apply about 1 ounce (2 tablespoons) of sunscreen to your entire body 30 minutes before going outside. Reapply every two hours or immediately after swimming or excessive sweating. Make sure to apply to all exposed areas. Don't forget your ears, neck, scalp, hands, feet, and ankles. Re-apply to all exposed areas every two hours or as directed on the sunscreen packaging. Some sunscreens are waterproof for 80 minutes, so make sure to re-apply after swimming or sweating.
  - Examine your skin head-to-toe every month.
  - See your physician every year for a professional skin exam.

Some other helpful suggestions:

- Bring a large umbrella or umbrella chair if you know you'll be in the sun for long periods of time.
- Be aware that snow, sand, and water reflect UV rays and magnify their effect. This can increase your odds of getting sunburn and skin cancer.
- Ask your physician or pharmacist if any of your medications increase your sensitivity to the sun.
- Stay hydrated to avoid your skin drying out, which may make you more susceptible to burning.

Following these simple tips can help you to not only avoid skin cancer but keep your skin looking young and healthy. We'll study this idea more closely in the next chapter.

How to Keep Your Youthful Appearance

Lola crushes her cigarette into an ashtray and stares in the mirror. Is that really her? She recalls a time when her face was free of wrinkles and sunspots, but those days are almost a distant memory. Now she feels like the skin on her face resembles a Shar-pei. Years of heavy drinking, smoking, and sun worshiping have taken a toll. What has happened to her youthful appearance?

One of the most visible signs of aging is our skin condition. However, our skin does more than just make us worry about wrinkles and age spots. It serves many important functions, including protection, regulation, and sensation. Skin acts as a barrier, protecting us from injuries, temperature fluctuations, micro-organisms, and chemicals. It regulates our body temperature via sweating and hair. For example, the hairs on our arms lay flat when we are warm and rise when we are cold. Skin also allows for the synthesis of Vitamin D. Our skin contains many nerve cells and receptors that provide information about heat, cold, pain, and touch. Can you believe it's the largest organ in our body in terms of surface area and weight? For these reasons, it's important to take time out of our busy schedule to make sure we're doing our best to keep our skin healthy.

Ultraviolet light from the sun comes in the form of long wavelength ultraviolet A (UVA) and shortwave ultraviolet B (UVB) rays. They are a form of radiation, which means they can cause changes to the cells in our skin. UVA rays can penetrate deeply into our skin, potentially resulting in wrinkles and skin aging. UVB rays affect the outer layers of skin, causing sunburns, tans, and skin cancer. That's why sunscreen needs to protect against both types of rays.

Suntans and burns stimulate skin cells to quickly reproduce to promote healing. This hastened process can cause errors in cell reproduction, which may lead to skin cancer. One way we can keep our skin healthy is to take measures to try to prevent skin cancer as described previously.

How else can we keep our skin healthy? Our diet plays an important role. The nutrients in our food help our cells to replicate. Eating foods with antioxidants may help to decrease inflammation associated with skin damage. Examples include blueberries, raspberries, spinach, nuts, and seeds. A diet rich in Vitamin C may also aid skin health. A general rule of thumb is to eat a colorful variety of fruits and vegetables throughout the day.

When possible, try to eat organic fruits and vegetables to decrease exposure to harmful toxins. Most people are on a budget, and organic produce tends to be more expensive. The Environmental Working Group (EWG) has created a list called the "Clean 15 and the Dirty Dozen."[8] It highlights which fruits and vegetables have the lowest levels of pesticides and harmful chemicals and which are the most contaminated. If possible, buy organic foods listed among the Dirty Dozen. See Chapter 6 for further information.

A healthy diet with whole grains and lean proteins can promote skin health. Healthy fats, such as avocados, olive oil, flax seeds, nuts, and fish can be incorporated into your diet.

It's also important to stay hydrated. Aim to drink at least 48-64 ounces of water per day. Not drinking enough water can lead to dry, flaky skin, dry eyes, and less than optimal bodily functioning. For more information about hydration, please refer to Chapter 11.

Limit your sun exposure. Small amounts of sunlight are beneficial, allowing us to produce Vitamin D and improving our mood. However, use sunscreen as discussed above and wear sunglasses and sun hats.

When possible, avoid harsh chemicals by opting for natural skin products. The Environmental Working Group has created Skin Deep®, a cosmetic safety database.[9] Take advantage of its wealth of information and avoid exposing yourself to potentially harmful chemicals. Invest time by looking up each of the skincare products you use and reading about their safety, including possible concerns and health hazards.

Try to use non-toxic cleaning products. Harmful chemicals can be absorbed through the skin and breathed into your lungs. Non-toxic products are better for not only your skin, but your lungs and overall health. The EWG website also includes a database for cleaning products.[10]

One way you can decrease indoor pollution is to own plants. Plants provide us with critical oxygen. They help add moisture to the air. In addition, they filter harmful toxins from our environment. B.C. Wolverton's book How to Grow Fresh Air highlights fifty houseplants that can improve the air quality of your home and office.[11]

If you want younger looking skin and you smoke, consider quitting. Ask your physician for advice and assistance on how to kick the habit. Smoking decreases blood flow by constricting the blood vessels in the skin. This decreases oxygen and nutrient supply to the skin, thus impacting skin health. Smoking damages collagen and elastin, which are fibers that give your skin strength and elasticity. In addition, the frequent facial movements that some smokers make, such as lip pursing and eye squinting, can also lead to wrinkles.

Acne and skin problems aren't just for teenagers anymore. Stress can trigger acne breakouts and other skin issues. Take time to manage stress by using relaxation techniques such as meditation, managing your to-do list, setting aside time to do the things you enjoy, and exercising. Exercise also increases the circulation of oxygen and nutrients and releases toxins through perspiration.

Aim to get eight hours of quality sleep each night. Your skin rejuvenates and repairs itself while you're sleeping. For more about getting a good night's sleep, please refer to Chapter 22.

Treat your skin gently. Take warm (not hot) showers and baths to avoid removing too much oil from your skin. Use mild cleansers and check ingredient labels to avoid harsh chemicals. Take care when shaving to avoid unnecessary nicks and cuts. Shave in the direction the skin grows and not against it. Apply a moisturizer daily and try to use an SPF moisturizer as described above.

In summary, sunscreen, diet, hydration, skin products, cleaning products, smoking, stress, and sleep can all impact skin. By following the suggestions above, you can help keep your skin healthy throughout middle age and beyond.

Chapter 17

Your Immune System in Action

*R*oberta sneezes three times and reaches for a tissue. She just got over a cold two *weeks ago. Could she already be getting another one? She's had four bad colds in the last five months, not to mention a stomach bug and the flu. Is something wrong with her immune system?*

Have you ever heard people say they have a good immune system? Or perhaps they frequently get sick and complain that their immune system doesn't do its job. But what exactly is your immune system?

I'm a nationally certified lymphedema therapist (CLT-LANA). When I tell people that, I usually get a blank or confused look, followed by either "What kind of therapist?" or "What's lymphedema?" In a nutshell, I work with people who have a problem with their lymphatic system. One of the functions of this important system involves our immune response.

Your heart pumps out 100% of your blood throughout your body via arteries. Ninety percent of this blood returns to your heart through your veins. The other 10% returns to your heart as lymph fluid via your lymphatic system. Lymph fluid consists of proteins, water, red blood cells, leukocytes (white blood cells), waste products, and fat.

Lymph (also called lymphatic fluid) is absorbed into lymph capillaries from the extracellular spaces (also known as interstitium, or spaces between your cells). One of the main jobs of the lymphatic system is to transport proteins. In fact, about 75-100 grams of proteins are transported by the lymphatic system each day.

The immune system is a team of cells, tissues and organs that work together to protect the body. Leukocytes, also known as white blood cells, are found in organs such as the spleen and in bone marrow. One type of leukocyte is called a lymphocyte.

How does the lymphatic system affect your immune system? It transports lymphocytes, cancer cells, cell debris, and bacteria. In the small intestines, cholesterol, fat-soluble vitamins A, D, E, and K, and long chain triglycerides are absorbed into the lymphatic system.

Lymph nodes are small organs within the lymphatic system. If you've ever had a sore throat, someone may have felt the sides of your neck and said you have "swollen glands." Although people sometimes refer to these lymph nodes as glands, this is incorrect because they do not secrete substances (like glands do).

There are approximately 600 to 700 lymph nodes in the human body. Most are in the abdomen, but there are also many in the head and neck region, axilla (armpit), and inguinal (groin) area. They range in size from 2 mm to 2.5 cm.

Lymph nodes have numerous functions. They filter bacteria, toxins, and dead cells. They produce white blood cells. White blood cells are very important to our immune system. They help to remove germs and fight infections. They also control the amount of proteins in the lymph and allow extra water to be reabsorbed by the body.

Sometimes, the immune system malfunctions or does not work the way it should. For example, a person may develop allergies. In this case, the immune system overreacts to a substance, such as pollen, ragweed, dust, dander, or foods like peanuts or tree nuts. People may also develop auto-immune conditions, such as rheumatoid arthritis or diseases like cancer.

How can you boost your immune system and help it to function at its very best?

- Wash your hands regularly. This is the single most effective way to get rid of germs and prevent infections. Carry a small container of hand sanitizer in your lunch bag or purse.
- Eat a healthy diet packed with nutritious foods, like fruits and vegetables.
- Get enough sleep. See Chapter 22 for specifics.
- Exercise regularly.
- Get regular well visits with your physician. See an allergist or immunologist if you have allergies or problems with your immune system.

By incorporating these steps into your lifestyle, you can help your immune system do its job effectively to keep you healthy.

Chapter 18

Strategies to Improve Balance and Prevent Falls

Candy Richards feels like she's been off-balance for the past year. Her physician sent her for a whole battery of tests, but they all came back negative. It has come to the point where she dares not leave her home without a cane because she is terrified of falling. She knows what happens to people who break their hips. Her friend Boris broke his last year, and now he lives in a nursing home.

Do you ever feel off balance? Or do you want to make sure you stay steady on your feet as you get older? Then this chapter is for you.

Good balance is necessary to reduce the risk of falls and subsequent injuries. The National Council on Aging (NCOA) shares some frightening statistics about falls.[1]

- One in four Americans over the age of sixty-five falls each year.
- Every 11 seconds, an older adult is treated in the emergency room for a fall, and every 19 minutes, one dies from a fall.
- Falls are the leading cause of fatal injury among older adults.
- Falls result in more than 2.8 million injuries treated in emergency departments annually, including over 800,000 hospitalizations and more than 27,000 deaths.

Our sense of balance allows us to know where our bodies are in space and to maintain a desired position. Our balance depends on information from our visual system (eyes), vestibular system (ears), and musculoskeletal system (proprioceptors found in our muscles and joints).

All three components work together in order to have and maintain normal balance.

Vestibular means relating to the inner ear. The inner ear makes up our sense of balance. The labyrinth consists of a hollow, bony cavity in the innermost part of the ear. It serves two functions: hearing and balance.

Our visual system also contributes to our sense of balance. It keeps objects from blurring when moving, such as when you are walking or riding in a car or standing on a platform at a train station when a train goes by. Vision keeps us aware of our position with movement. To best utilize our visual system for balance, we need light. That's why more people fall at night walking to the bathroom if it's dark: their visual component of balance has been taken away. Instead, people must then rely on muscles and the vestibular system to remain upright.

Skeletal muscles contribute to balance via proprioceptors (sensory receptors) found in tendons and muscle fibers. Proprioception assists us in maintaining the position of our body at rest or in motion. It provides us with our unconscious perception of movement and spatial orientation. For example, it includes the sense that your foot is on a step when you are going up and down stairs. The vestibular system works with the visual and vestibular systems to relay information to our brain to control our balance.

People can have both balance and dizziness disorders. A balance disorder, or disequilibrium, can occur after a stroke. A dizziness disorder, such as benign paroxysmal positional vertigo (BPPV), stems from the ear. According to the American Physical Therapy Association, a balance disorder is a "fleeting sense of spinning." Forty percent of Americans will experience an episode of dizziness leading to a doctor's visit. Balance disorders are generally caused by certain health disorders and inner ear problems. Our sense of balance may decline as we age because our muscles may weaken, our visual system may lose acuity, and our vestibular system may decline.

There are many reasons for balance impairments. General causes include ear infections (viral/bacterial), neurological disorders, blood circulation disorders (such as a decrease in blood pressure), and certain medications. For example, chemotherapy can cause chemotherapy induced peripheral neuropathy. This nerve damage can affect sensation and strength, thus impacting balance. Likewise, sleeping pills and muscle relaxants can affect balance.

Balance impairments can be due to neurological disorders. Transient ischemic attacks (also called TIA or mini stroke) and cerebrovascular accidents (stroke) can cause weakness and affect the balance center of the brain, called the cerebellum. Multiple sclerosis leads to weakness, decreased balance, and increased risk of falls. Parkinson's disease can lead to problems with balance. Parkinson's disease also affects posture; people have a shuffling gait which can cause tripping. Likewise, head injuries, such as traumatic brain injury, can impair balance.

Patients with diabetes can experience a decrease in balance due to diabetic neuropathy. Neuropathy involves dysfunction of peripheral nerves, resulting in symptoms such as numbness, burning, and weakness. This can impair sensation and movement, especially in the feet. Musculoskeletal disorders such as faulty posture, orthopedic surgeries, and decreased strength in the legs and/or trunk muscles can also contribute to poor balance.

Vestibular disorders such as benign paroxysmal positional vertigo (BPPV) affect crystals in the inner ear. They cause a person to feel like the room is spinning, which is called vertigo. Sometimes people use the terms vertigo and dizziness interchangeably, but they are not exactly the same. Dizziness is a term that includes sensations such as lightheadedness, feeling faint, weak, unsteady, or woozy. Dizziness can be caused by a multitude of conditions, such as low blood pressure, low blood sugar, anxiety, stress, and migraines. People with vertigo will feel off-balance and have the sensation that the room is spinning; it is a false sensation of movement. In addition, they may experience nausea and vomiting. People with BPPV can be helped by ear-nose-throat specialists (ENTs) and physical therapists specializing in vertigo.

As people age, muscular-skeletal, neuro-muscular, and postural changes occur. Arthritic changes occur in the neck, trunk, hips, and knees and can affect range of motion and mobility. Osteoarthritis can affect walking patterns and balance, thereby leading to an increased risk of falls. Neuromuscular changes may occur with aging. These changes result in problems with mobility, coordination, proprioception (body in space), pain and weakness.

People with a minor balance problem may not necessarily fall. It's important to stay strong and active to decrease fall risk.

Balance Evaluation

Poor balance may not be due to a specific diagnosis. It can be related to a nonspecific degenerative process (such as arthritis) that's influenced by genetics, activity level, socio-economic factors, personality, education, and undiagnosed disease.

Changes in your musculoskeletal and neuromuscular system can affect your balance. For example, poor posture can be caused by a lifetime of slouching, improper lifting, or a desk job. Faulty posture can impact gait (walking) patterns, leading to poor balance. Normal walking velocity is one meter per second. People with slow gait patterns may have trouble with turning, going to the bathroom, or even crossing the road.

Your nervous system allows messages to be sent from your brain through neurons to tell muscles what to do. With age, the synapses or connections decrease and may cause your muscles to get weak. Decreased activity level leads to decreased mobility. You need to move, walk, and do exercises to keep your heart healthy so that it can pump blood which is rich in oxygen to all your muscles. A good supply of oxygen leads to healthy tissue.

It's a good idea to review your medications yearly with your doctor or pharmacist and ask about their side effects. Sleeping pills, antidepressants, allergy/cold/flu medications, and painkillers can make you feel drowsy, which could affect balance. Medications for seizure disorders, Parkinson's disease, and diabetes may result in dizziness. Medications for high blood pressure can also cause dizziness if they make your blood pressure too low. Diuretics can make you rush to the toilet, increasing fall risk.

Periodic checkups of your ears are recommended because they're important for both hearing and balance. We rely on our sense of sound for orientation to the environment that surrounds us. If you have decreased hearing, you might not be as quickly aware of a potentially hazardous situation. For example, hearing sounds such as cars or running water gives a clue as to what is around you.

Vision is one of the three systems to help us maintain normal balance. As we age, visual acuity decreases. Visual acuity is the ability to read numbers and letters at a given distance. There's also a decline in depth perception. Depth perception is the ability to judge distances and spaces among objects. For example, you may turn around to sit in a chair but miss. Perhaps you misjudge ascending or descending stairs/curbs. Or, while driving, you nearly hit another car or pedestrian due to poor depth perception. Carpets with busy patterns, stairs, and curbs can become risk factors for increasing fall risk.

The ability to adjust to sudden changes in light (brightness or darkness) can also be affected by aging. It may take longer for eyes to accommodate. Wearing glasses or contacts with old prescriptions can alter visual field, which can affect balance. Conditions like glaucoma or cataracts can limit vision as well. It's recommended to have your eyes checked at least once a year or if there is a sudden change in vision.

In addition to the internal factors above, there are also external factors that affect your balance. These may include:

- Poor lighting: You need proper lighting, especially in the bedroom, bathroom, and entranceways.
- Home/outside environment: Use railings on indoor/outside stairs. Utilize grab bars in the bathroom as needed.
- Flooring, uneven rugs/carpets: If throw rugs are slippery, get rid of them or secure them with a reliable non-skid backing.
- Pets: You may trip over small pets or large ones may knock you down.
- Uneven surfaces: These may include curbs or uneven sidewalks. Always wear good shoes with non-skid soles.
- Weather: Rain, snow, and ice can cause slippery conditions.

Symptoms of balance disorders are unique to each individual. They may include:

- Difficulty remaining upright (vertical)
- Vertigo/spinning/feeling of dizziness
- Difficulty moving in and out of positions quickly (For example, in the case of BPPV, crystals dislodge from the inner ear, leading to vertigo and impaired balance).
- Hearing loss/tinnitus (ringing in the ears)
- Numbness in the legs (may be due to nerve involvement or blood clots)
- Two or more falls in the last year

Balance problems may be difficult to describe for individuals. They may have a gradual onset or may occur quickly due to a traumatic event. If you feel you have a balance disorder, it's important to contact a physician to assess your problem.

Balance profoundly affects our ability to function. Fear of falling may cause one to become sedentary. Inactivity can lead to increased weakness. A decrease in function may include trouble taking care of oneself, walking, cooking, or getting around. If the doctor diagnoses you with a balance disorder, you may be referred for a physical therapy evaluation. The assessment includes:

- Reviewing your past medical history, falls history, and medication list
- Measuring strength
- Evaluating gait (walking pattern)
- Assessing balance and fall risk with various tests, such as the Timed Up and Go (TUG), single limb stance, the Tinetti Balance and Gait Assessment, and Double stance/tandem stance (Romberg/Sharpened Romberg). Please refer to Appendix B for a sample balance screening tool for balance screening.
  - The TUG requires a person to stand up from a chair with armrests, walk 10 feet, turn around, walk back to their chair, and sit down. A time greater than or equal to 14 seconds indicates an increased risk for falling. Greater than or equal to 30 seconds indicates that you may need an assistive device to help you walk more safely.
  - Single limb stance tests your ability to balance on one foot without upper extremity support (without holding onto something with your hands). You should be able to stand on one foot for at least 5 seconds to lessen fall risk.
  - Tinetti Balance and Gait Assessment assesses a variety of activities related to balance and gait, such as standing up, sitting down, turning around, and quality of gait pattern.
  - Double stance/tandem stance (Romberg/Sharpened Romberg): Double stance means two feet close together and tandem means one foot in front of the other, such that the toes of one foot touch the heel of the other. The test is performed

with eyes open as well as closed. If your eyes are closed, you must use a system other than visual to maintain your balance.

Fall Prevention Tips

Some falls are avoidable. For example, non-skid mats could help prevent needless falls in showers and tubs. Likewise, taking the time to tack down or put non-skid backing on throw rugs could also prevent unnecessary injuries.

It's a good idea to find a few minutes to take a close look around your home. Here are some steps you can take to make your house safer and decrease your risk of falling.

- Make sure you have a clear path to walk around your house. Remove clutter and things that you can trip over (paper, books, clothes, shoes, etc.) from stairs and places you walk through the house.
- Remove throw rugs or use double sided tape/non-slip backing so rugs won't slide.
- Remove loose cords that could cause one to trip.
- Make sure wires from lamps, telephones, and extension cords are next to walls so you can't trip over them.
- Keep halls, entries, and stairways well lit. Use night lights in hallways and bathrooms.
- Get up slowly from lying down or sitting to avoid dizziness. Keep a flashlight with fresh batteries by your bedside.
- Use assistive devices such as canes, walkers, or long handled reachers as needed.
- Wear shoes with non-skid soles. Avoid wearing loose fitting slippers that could make you slip.

STAIRS

- Fix uneven or loose steps; ensure carpet is firmly attached to each step.
- Use railings on stairs and escalators.
- If possible, have handrails on both sides of the staircase both inside and outside of the home.
- Keep steps free from clutter.
- Have adequate lighting in the stairway.

KITCHEN

- Move items you use often to lower shelves.
- Use a sturdy step stool if necessary.
- Use non-skid rubber mats near the sink and stove in the kitchen.

BATHROOMS

- Use a non-slip rubber mat on the floor of the tub/shower.
- Install grab bars near the toilet and in the shower to help get in and out.
- Consider using a shower tub seat if necessary.
- You can use a raised toilet seat if you have trouble standing.

BEDROOMS

- Make sure a lamp is near your bed and easy to reach.
- Ensure the path from bedroom to bathroom is well lit. Use a nightlight if necessary.
- Keep a flashlight close by in case of power outages.

OTHER

- Be sure to have your vision checked on a regular basis.
- Request your doctor or pharmacist review your medications to see if any cause drowsiness or dizziness, which can increase fall risk.
- Limit the amount of alcohol you drink, as it can impair balance and judgment.

- When you get out of bed, sit on the side of the bed for several minutes before standing up. This allows your blood pressure time to adjust.
- Get screened for osteoporosis.
- If your doctor gives you medical clearance, begin an exercise program. It can make you stronger and improve your balance. Now, let's check out some balance exercises you can incorporate into your routine.

Balance Exercises

Are you ready to start improving your balance? When performing balance exercises, make sure not to stand in the middle of a room. It's a good idea to keep a chair behind you in case you lose your balance and need to sit down quickly. You should have support close by, such as two sturdy chairs or a kitchen counter. If you use a walker, you can use that as your support.

Since good balance is partially dependent upon sight, focusing on a single, stationary object will help you to maintain better standing balance.

To improve your balance, aim to perform the balance exercises below 3 to 5 days per week.

Heel and toe raise: While standing, raise up on your toes as you lift your heels off the ground. Then rock back on your heels, making sure your toes are off the floor. Make sure to stand near a stable object to hold if needed. Repeat 10 to 20 times. *Please refer to Figures 21-22.*

Single leg standing: Stand on one leg and maintain your balance. Alternate standing on one foot for 5-10 seconds, then the other foot for 5-10 seconds. Make sure your legs are not touching. Stand near a stable object, like a countertop or back of a sturdy chair, so that you can hold on for support if needed. Hold on as little as possible but as much as necessary. Repeat 3 to 5 times on each leg.

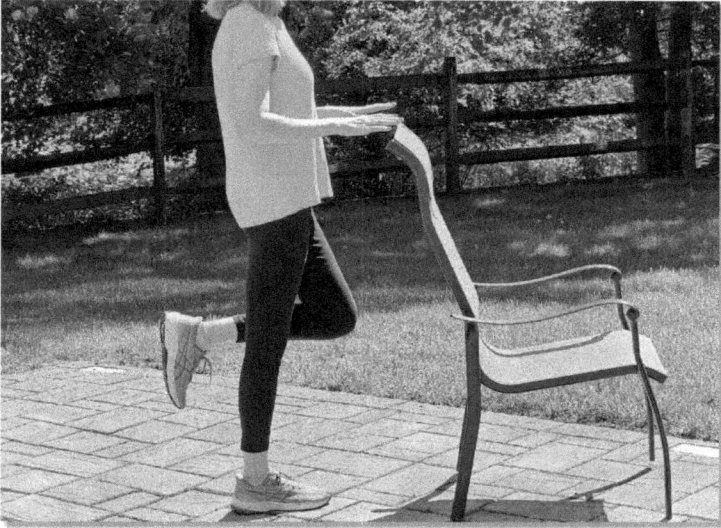

Figure 57 Single leg standing

Heel-toe walking: Walk forwards with a "heel-toe" walking pattern (the heel of the foot in front touches the toe of the foot behind). Pretend you are walking on a tightrope. Make sure to walk near a stable object such as a kitchen counter so that you can hold on if needed.

Tandem stance: Stand next to a sturdy chair, table, or countertop for support. Hold on as little as possible but as much as necessary. Place the heel of your right foot so that it is touching the toes of your left foot. Both feet should be pointing straight ahead. Balance in this position for 5-10 seconds. Switch feet and repeat with your left foot in front of right. Repeat 3-5 times.

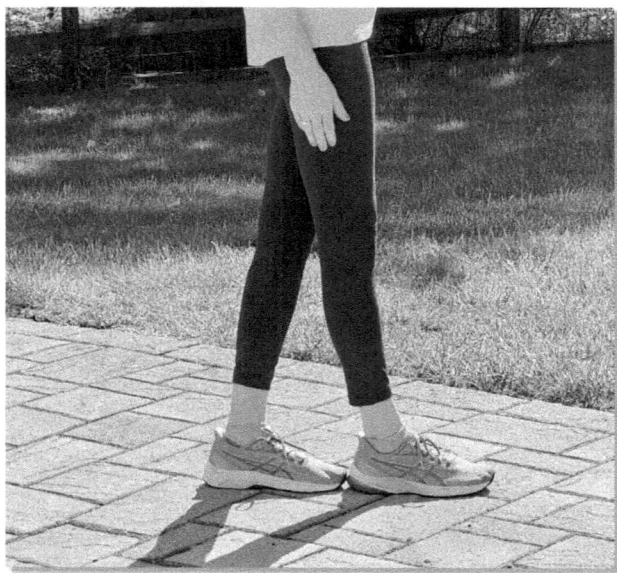

Figure 58 Tandem stance

Marching in place: Alternate lifting each knee high as you march in place. Hold on to a countertop or the back of a sturdy chair if needed. Repeat 10 to 20 times. You can add a strengthening component to this balance exercise by adding ankle weights. *Please refer to Figure 17.*

Sidestepping: Walk sideways (hold onto a countertop as needed). Alternate stepping to the left and then to the right.

Static standing (Romberg): Stand next to a chair, table, or countertop for support if needed. Stand with your feet together and your arms across your chest while keeping your balance with your eyes open. Do the same exercise with your eyes closed to make it more challenging. Begin with your feet shoulder width apart and progress to feet together.

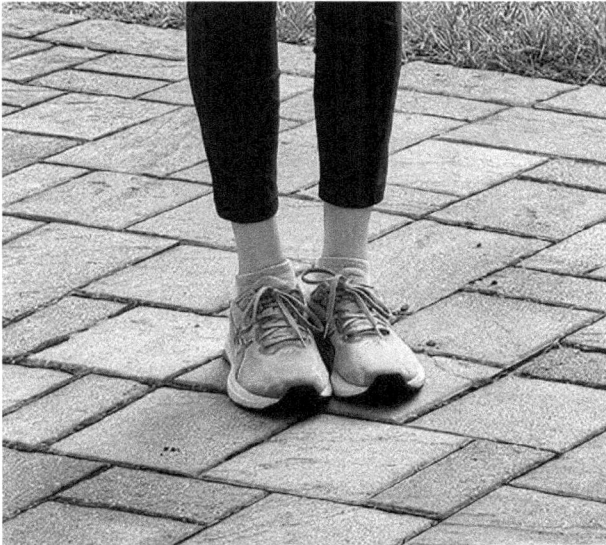

Figure 59 Static standing with feet together (Romberg)

Chapter 19

The Effects of Stress and Coping Strategies

Ellie looks at the pile of work on her desk and swears she can practically feel her blood pressure rising. Her head begins pounding and her stomach feels like it is tied in knots. She's never been able to meet her deadlines. If she doesn't quit her job, she feels like all this stress will either give her a heart attack or a stroke.

If you are like most Americans, you often feel some sort of stress. According to the American Psychological Association Stress in America Report, 42% of Americans lie awake at night due to stress and 20 percent report episodes of extreme stress in their lives.[1,2] But what exactly is stress?

Stress is our response to environmental pressures. These responses can be physical, emotional, or mental in nature. Stress is a normal part of life. Depending on the circumstances, it can be good or bad. What happens when you "get stressed?" The autonomic nervous system controls many autonomic processes in the body, such as heart rate, blood pressure, breathing rate, temperature, and digestion. Your hypothalamus, a part of your brain which is the main control center for your autonomic nervous system, sends out a message to your body to release the hormones (cortisol and adrenaline). These trigger the body's "fight or flight" response. You may feel your breathing rate increase, your heart rate quicken, and your muscles tense as they prepare for action.

Acute stress produces the "fight or flight" response. It creates a burst of energy that helps you deal with emergency situations. This could be something as simple as your response to a scary amusement park ride or your reaction to barely avoiding a car accident. Maybe you hear a strange noise and worry there could be a burglar in your home. This type of stress

206

is not bad for your health. Rather, it helps you to deal with stressful situations.

If stress lasts for long periods of time, it's called chronic stress. Being in a constant state of "preparedness" can adversely affect your body. It can be a factor in heart and lung disease, cancer, and mental health. It can cause headaches, dizziness, anxiety, digestive disorders, and other problems.

What one perceives to be stressful may be exciting and exhilarating for another. Are you the kind of person who would be thrilled to perform on stage or would you experience stage fright? Stress can be good, such as when you give birth to a child or win an award. Other times, the effects of stress can be detrimental to your health.

The Negative Effects of Stress

People often blame illness for headaches, stomach pains, or trouble sleeping. However, stress may be the culprit. Chronic stress can be responsible for all these symptoms, as well as muscle pain or tension, chest pain, fatigue, or altered sex drive.

Stress doesn't just impact us physically. It can affect mood, leading to irritability, anxiety, and depression. People under chronic stress may feel restlessness and may find it difficult to focus.

In addition, chronic stress can affect behavior, leading to over or undereating. People may be more likely to turn to drugs, alcohol, or tobacco. Chronic stress can lead to social withdrawal and isolation. In addition, people who are suffering from stress tend to be less likely to exercise.

Since stress hormones increase respiratory rate, they can make it harder for someone with lung diseases such as asthma or emphysema to breathe. They also affect the cardiovascular system because they increase heart rate and constrict blood vessels. This sends more oxygen to the muscles, but the result is an increase in blood pressure. If it occurs frequently, it can lead to an increased risk of heart attack and stroke.

Stress hormones can also cause acid reflux and heartburn. Stress impacts the speed with which food travels along the digestive system. It may speed it up, leading to diarrhea. Alternatively, it may slow it down, resulting in constipation. It can also cause nausea, vomiting, and stomachache. Stress increases the risk of developing diabetes because your liver produces extra glucose (blood sugar) to give you a boost of energy. If your body cannot manage this extra glucose, type 2 diabetes may develop.

People who are under chronic stress may not relax their muscles. This may lead to muscle pain, such as neck and back pain, and headaches.

Ongoing stress can inhibit sexual desire. For women, stress can cause irregular, heavier, or more painful periods. It may also exacerbate the physical symptoms of menopause. For men, chronic stress can cause testosterone levels to drop, leading to decreased sperm production as well as possible erectile dysfunction or impotence.

Chronic stress can make you more susceptible to catching viral illnesses such as a cold or the flu by weakening your immune system. It can also lengthen your recovery time from illness. People can become so used to stress that they become numb to it. They are so accustomed to stress that they perceive it as normal. Fortunately, there are things you can do to decrease the effects of stress. Keep reading to learn more about what you can do to manage stress.

What is "Diaphragmatic Breathing"?

The diaphragm is a dome-shaped muscle that forms the floor of the rib cage. Even though it is the most efficient muscle for breathing and relaxation, many people are not familiar with using it. It helps to regulate pressures in the thoracic and abdominal cavities, which can affect everything from balance to speech and eating.

Diaphragmatic breathing, also called belly breathing, is an important technique to learn because it helps relax and settle down the autonomic nervous system. When belly breathing, the diaphragm moves downward during inhalation and upward during exhalation. The correct use of diaphragmatic breathing can help quiet brain activity resulting in relaxation of the muscles and organs of the body. This is accomplished by slow rhythmic breathing concentrated in the diaphragm muscle rather than the chest.

Diaphragmatic breathing has numerous benefits. It promotes relaxation and may help you to fall asleep. It can be used as a urinary urge control technique, helping you gain better control of your bladder. Since it is an efficient muscle for breathing, it's of particular benefit to people with lung problems, such as chronic obstructive pulmonary disease (COPD). It can decrease oxygen demand and lessen the work of breathing. In addition, diaphragmatic breathing stimulates your lymphatic system.

Last year, I was treating a woman with urinary incontinence. She had a history of stroke five years earlier, and reported she had "dragged her left leg" ever since. By utilizing simple physical therapy techniques to facilitate her diaphragm on her weaker side, she was able to greatly improve her walking pattern.

How to Perform Diaphragmatic Breathing

Start by lying on your back with your head supported and a pillow under your knees. Alternatively, you can sit in a recliner in a relaxed position. Place one hand on your upper chest and the other on your abdomen (just below your rib cage). This hand will allow you to feel the movement of the diaphragm as you breathe in and out. Relax your jaw by placing your tongue on the roof of your mouth and keeping your teeth slightly apart. Breathe in through your nose, letting your abdomen (belly) expand and rise while you keep your upper chest, neck and shoulders relaxed. You should feel your belly move into your hand. The hand on your belly should rise higher than the hand on your chest.

As you breathe out through your mouth, allow your abdomen and chest to fall. Exhale completely. The hand on your belly should now move inwards. Remember to breathe slowly. Don't force your breathing. Your breaths shouldn't be deeper or faster than normal breaths, as this may cause you to experience tingling in your hands and feet from hyperventilating.

Practice this exercise for five minutes several times per day. If you're still having trouble locating your diaphragm, place your hand just below your rib cage and take a few quick sniffs. You should feel the diaphragm jump into your hand. This is the muscle you are trying to harness for diaphragmatic breathing. As the diaphragm muscle becomes stronger, this exercise will become easier.

Relaxation Strategies

Jenna Bridges knows she is part of the "sandwich" generation. She is so stressed; she feels as if her stomach is tied in knots half the time. Her father had a major stroke two months ago and is in a rehab facility. Her mother has early-onset dementia, and Jenna worries about her living alone without someone to care for her. Her parents-in-law aren't faring much better. Her mother-in-law needs open heart surgery, and her father-in-law is battling prostate cancer. Her husband was recently laid off from his job as a chef, so Jenna is working extra hours at the deli to make ends meet. Her son is starting to apply to colleges, and her daughter is in drug rehab because she is addicted to painkillers after hurting her lower back playing soccer. Jenna knows she should take a few minutes to relax, but she isn't sure how to go about it. Lately, she is starting to feel like her heart is palpitating. She is beginning to think all this stress is going to be the death of her.

Stress is accepted as a part of life, and some people may not even recognize when they're under stress. They get used to a certain level of stress and perceive it as normal. Similarly, you may have excess muscle tension and not realize it. The tension has been there for so long that your body accepts it as normal, which makes it difficult to determine if the muscle is relaxed or tense. If this is the case, you may benefit from biofeedback with a healthcare provider to help you learn how to relax your muscles.

Tense muscles may cause or perpetuate pain. Excessive tension in muscles restricts blood flow. This can irritate the muscles, causing pain and more tension. Learning how to relax the muscles helps to break the pain pattern and promotes recovery.

In attempting to relax, it's helpful to learn to determine the difference between relaxed and contracted. At first, it may be difficult to distinguish the difference, since it's hard to describe and there may not be a big difference between the two states. Be persistent and pay close attention to how the muscle feels. The following is a list of helpful hints.

- Rely on yourself (not others) to manage your care. No one knows your body or how you are feeling better than you do. You are your own best advocate. However, seek help if you're under unmanageable stress. Physicians, social workers, psychologists, therapists, self-help groups, clergy members, and books can help you learn how to deal with stress effectively. Don't feel like you have to figure it out all on your own.

- Set aside some time for yourself. Don't wait until someone tells you to relax. Instead, take the initiative and make it a priority.

- Avoid being in one position for too long. Make sure to move and stretch during the day.

There are many different relaxation methods available. Try several different ones to determine which works best for you. If possible, try relaxing for 20-30 minutes per day. Relaxing is a skill that takes practice. Keep working at it until you can relax quickly and completely.

Specific Relaxation Techniques

- Create a quiet environment with dim lights and a comfortable temperature. Make yourself comfortable, but don't fall asleep.

- Diaphragmatic breathing promotes relaxation by calming your autonomic nervous system. Take a slow breath through your nose, allowing your abdomen (belly) to expand and rise. Exhale slowly through your mouth, allowing your belly to fall. This type of breathing should be relaxed and gentle, not forced. Please see a detailed description of how to perform diaphragmatic breathing above.

- Visualization techniques facilitate relaxation. Imagine you are in a quiet, relaxing place such as the mountains or an empty beach. What do you see? Smell? Hear? Make your quiet place as real as possible.

- Body Scanning is a technique in which periodically throughout the day, you stop and bring your attention to various parts of the body (eyes, cheeks, jaw, head, neck, shoulders, arms, hands, ribs, belly, buttock, legs, and feet). Check each area for tension and pause to allow the tension to leave your body.

- Guided Imagery is a method of focused relaxation. It uses visualization and imagination to promote relaxation and improved health. People often choose to use a therapist or cell phone app to practice this technique. In essence, a person finds a quiet place to relax and be comfortable. First, use diaphragmatic breathing as above to help relax. Then, clear all the thoughts from your mind and imagine something using all your senses (vision, hearing, touch, taste, smell). For example, imagine that you are in your favorite place or a place you would like to be. What do you see? What sounds do you hear? Can you feel anything around you? Are you eating or drinking in this place? If yes, what does it taste like? What do you smell? Relax and use your imagination for 10-20 minutes.

- Mindful Meditation allows the mind to block out "chatter" and focus on what the body is doing. In this way, one can enter a more calm and focused state of being. The following are some simple steps to try.

1. Find a quiet, comfortable place where you will not be disturbed. It can be inside or outside, whichever you prefer.
2. Sit or lie down and keep your back straight (but not stiff). Use a pillow to support your head and neck as needed.
3. Focus on the present as you dismiss thoughts of the past or future.
4. Perform diaphragmatic breathing as described above. Breath in through your nose and let your belly rise. Exhale through your mouth and let your belly fall. Notice the sensation of the air moving in and out of your body as you breathe.
5. Become aware of your thoughts and pay attention as they come and go. Pretend you are an outside observer as you take note of your thoughts. What are they about? Regardless of whether your thoughts are filled with worry, anxiety, fear, or hope, try to remain calm and simply take note of them.
6. If you find yourself getting lost in your thoughts, simply return to your breathing.
7. Begin to let each of your thoughts float away. Gradually let your mind become empty of thoughts. Focus on your breathing.
8. If thoughts return to your mind, gently send them away.
9. Allow yourself to stay calm like this for 10-20 minutes. As you prepare to end your session of mindful meditation, sit for a minute or two as you regain awareness of where you are.

There are numerous apps available to assist with mindfulness. If you prefer personal training, integrative medicine and wellness centers can assist you.

Chapter 20

Understanding the Basics of Cancer

*T*aylor first felt a lump in her right armpit a month ago while showering. She waited a few weeks, hoping it would go away on its own. When it didn't, she reluctantly made an appointment with her gynecologist. Her doctor promptly referred her for a mammogram. She grew concerned when they called her to come back for additional imaging. The mammogram looked suspicious in the area where she felt the lump. An ultrasound and biopsy confirmed her fear: she had breast cancer, just like her mother and sister.

According to USAFacts, a nonprofit that compiles government data, almost 40% of Americans will receive a diagnosis of cancer during their lifetime. Cancer, a word most of us never want to hear, is becoming a chronic disease. That means there are more and more cancer survivors walking among us. In fact, there are currently more than ten million survivors of cancer in the United States. According to the American Cancer Society, sixty-four percent of those diagnosed with cancer today will still be alive in five years. [1] The five-year cancer survival rate rose from 63.5% in 2000 to 68.4% in 2015. Between 2000 and 2019, the incidence rate (the rate of new cancer cases per 100,000 people) decreased by 5.4%. During this same period, the annual mortality rate fell by more than 26%. These statistics are great reasons for hope, but cancer-related disabilities are the number one source of activity and participation restrictions. More people are surviving cancer diagnoses, but the cancer itself and cancer treatments such as chemotherapy and radiation can cause numerous side effects.

Seventh-grade science class is probably a distant memory, so let's do a quick refresher. Normal cells have certain characteristics. Each cell has 23 pairs of chromosomes. DNA is the genetic blueprint within the cells (i.e., our "genes").

Cells can undergo mutations, which are changes in the DNA sequence of a cell. In some cases, mutations may be caused by mistakes when cells divide. In other cases, they occur by exposure to DNA-damaging agents in the environment. This is a booming area in cancer research.

Although mutations can be harmful and lead to cancer or other diseases, they may at times be beneficial or have no effect. If they occur in cells that make eggs or sperm, they can be inherited.

Basic Cancer Terminology

Have you ever heard someone ask if a tumor is malignant or benign? The word benign usually elicits a giant sigh of relief. Benign neoplasms are non-cancerous tumors. In contrast, malignant neoplasms are cancerous tumors. They are composed of abnormal cells which grow and invade surrounding tissue. They have the ability to metastasize (spread to other areas of your body). "Primary site" indicates the body part where the tumor originates.

There are more than 100 types of cancer. Common ones include carcinoma, sarcoma, leukemia, lymphoma, myeloma, and central nervous system (CNS) neoplasms. Cancer is named according to the tissue of origin. It's an unregulated growth of abnormal cells. Cancer may present as changes (mutations) in your DNA (genetic makeup). Unfortunately, if cancer is left unchecked, it can spread to other body parts.

People facing a diagnosis of cancer often ask what caused it. There's no easy answer. Cancer development is due to many factors. Complex mechanisms cause changes in oncogenes, which are genes that cause a normal cell to transform into a cancerous one. In addition, genetic and environmental factors play a role. External agents like chemicals can interact with genetics, resulting in cancer. For example, lung cancer is often attributed to chemicals, skin cancer to ultraviolet rays, and cervical cancer to viruses.

Sometimes, cancer may be unavoidable. However, you can try to reduce your risk by not smoking, eating healthy (organic when possible), staying active, avoiding excessive ultraviolet rays, and wearing sunscreen to name just a few. If you are or a loved one is facing a cancer diagnosis, take comfort in the knowledge that you are not alone. Exciting advances in the treatment of cancer provide hope for the future.

The American Academy of Sports Medicine Moving through Cancer initiative compiled evidence about the "Effects of Exercise on Health-Related Outcomes in Those with Cancer." They found strong evidence to support aerobic exercise and resistance exercises for cancer-related fatigue, health-related quality of life, physical function, anxiety, depression, and lymphedema. They found moderate evidence to support exercise for bone health and sleep.

According to the 2018 Physical Activity Guidelines for Americans, 150-300 min/week of moderate exercise or 75-150 min/week of vigorous aerobic exercise can help with the prevention of seven common cancers (bladder, breast, colon, endometrial, esophageal, kidney, and stomach cancers) and the survival of three common cancers (breast, colon, and prostate). The exact dose is unknown, but overall, more exercise leads to better risk reduction. In summary, avoid inactivity, and to improve general health, aim to achieve the current physical activity guidelines for health (150 min /week aerobic exercise and 2x/week strength training). Exercise is medicine!

I am a PORi-certified oncology rehabilitation therapist. I work in an outpatient setting with patients recovering from breast cancer, head and neck cancer, gynecologic cancers, blood cancers, and many other types. If you or a loved one is recovering from cancer, know that there are avenues to help you, such as rehab settings like mine to help with physical recovery, mental health specialists to ease emotional burdens, and countless non-profit organizations to help with financial burdens.

Part V: Wellness: Healthy Body, Healthy Spirit, and a Healthy Mind

Chapter 21

Keep Your Brain Active

*B*oris *turns on his blinker and pulls over to the side of the road. He hates admitting it, but he is lost. The frightening part is that he's driven on this road numerous times. Now what once seemed friendly and familiar seems dark and sinister. He'll have to use his navigation system to figure out how to get home.*

Have you ever walked into a room to get something or do something, but once you are there, you can't recall what it is that you want to do? Everyone has moments in which they forget where they put their keys or forget someone's name. These occasional memory lapses are common and usually nothing to worry about.

Dementia. It's a word that strikes fear in the hearts of many. Most people know at least one person who has dementia. But exactly what is it? Dementia is a loss of cognitive abilities that interferes with memory, thinking/reasoning, and behavior. It gradually worsens over time and interrupts one's ability to perform activities of daily living.

Becoming old doesn't cause dementia, but the risk increases with age. Other risk factors include family history and genetics.

Currently, it's estimated that 5.5 million Americans have dementia associated with Alzheimer's disease. The Alzheimer's Association shares some statistics about Alzheimer's disease.[1]

- Ten percent of people over the age of 65 have the disease.
- It's the sixth leading cause of death in the United States (it kills more people than breast cancer and prostate cancer combined).

- Every 66 seconds, someone in the United States develops the disease.
- Since 2000, deaths by cardiac disease have decreased by 14%, yet deaths from Alzheimer's disease have increased by 89%.
- In 2017, dementia cost our nation 259 billion in healthcare and long-term care costs.
- It's estimated that there will be about 16 million people in the United States with Alzheimer's dementia by the year 2050.

Dementia is often due to diseases such as Alzheimer's disease (60-80% of all cases) or multi-infarct dementia (a series of strokes that decrease blood supply to the brain and lead to impaired brain function). Other possible causes of dementia include Parkinson's disease, Huntington's disease, head trauma, and long-term abuse of alcohol or drugs.

Dementia tends to develop gradually over months or even years. A normal brain has more than 100 billion nerve cells, called neurons. They interconnect to communicate with each other, forming complex networks. In the case of Alzheimer's disease, nerve cells in the brain become damaged and are no longer able to perform their jobs. An early sign of Alzheimer's disease is trouble recalling newly learned information. Other signs and symptoms of dementia include memory loss, impaired ability to plan and for abstract thinking, and language disturbances. People with dementia may have altered judgment and may exhibit behavioral changes. They may show restlessness and suffer from sleep disturbances.

Dementia can be easily confused with delirium. In fact, delirium often occurs in patients with dementia. However, delirium differs because it tends to have an acute (rapid) onset and lasts for days to weeks. The person has altered consciousness and impaired attention span. They may have delusions and hallucinations.

One cause of delirium is infections. In my volunteer work as an emergency medical technician, we are sometimes dispatched for a "person with an altered mental status." Upon our arrival, we find our patient to be confused and disoriented. Later, we may learn the person was suffering from a urinary tract infection. Delirium can also be due to trauma, medications, and alcohol/drug use. The presence of delirium is a medical emergency. Unlike dementia, it is usually reversible with proper medical treatment.

Everyone has memory lapses at times. However, significant memory loss is not part of normal aging. The Alzheimer's Association (https//alz.org) provides ten early warning signs and symptoms of dementia.[1]

1. Memory loss that disrupts daily life
2. Challenges in planning or solving problems
3. Difficulty completing familiar tasks at home, at work, or at leisure
4. Confusion with time or place
5. Trouble understanding visual images and spatial relationships
6. New problems with words in speaking or writing
7. Misplacing things and losing the ability to retrace steps
8. Decreased or poor judgment
9. Withdrawal from work or physical activities
10. Changes in mood and personality

If you notice that you or a loved one is suffering from memory loss or other cognitive issues, consult your doctor. There are some risk factors you can't control, such as age, genetics, and family history. However, there are numerous ways you can keep your mind sharp as you age. Here are a few ideas:

1. **Start (or keep) writing!** I don't mean that you need to write a novel. Writing may include emails to friends and family. You

could even keep a daily journal of reflections or write about your past vacations.

2. **Read:** This allows you to learn new information and stimulates building new brain connections.

3. **Healthy eating:** It's been linked to brain health. A study by Michelle Luciano, et al demonstrated that older people who followed a Mediterranean diet retained more brain volume over a three-year period than those who did not follow the diet as closely.[2]

4. **Control blood pressure and cholesterol:** Use healthy eating, exercise, and, if necessary, medication to keep your blood pressure and cholesterol within acceptable ranges.

5. **Keep off excess pounds:** A study by Dr. W.L. Xu, et al found that both being overweight as well as obesity at mid-life independently increased the risk of getting dementia (both Alzheimer's disease as well as vascular dementia) later in life.[3]

6. **Solve puzzles:** Try solving a daily crossword puzzle. If that's not your cup of tea, there are numerous websites and magazines that specialize in brain teasers and puzzles. A study by R.S. Wilson, et al showed that performing mentally stimulating activities appears to slow cognitive decline before dementia onset in older adults.[4]

7. **Play board games or cards:** These activities engage the brain and stimulate thinking. Join your friends for bridge or rummy cube or settle down for a cozy game of solitaire.

8. **Sketch, draw, and paint:** These activities promote planning and artistic creativity.

9. **Play a musical instrument:** Have you always wanted to play the guitar, but never had the time or opportunity to learn? Retirement may provide the time to take up new hobbies, such as learning how to play the piano, harmonica, violin, or other musical instrument. If you can't play or are unable to learn, don't despair. Research shows that even listening to music is beneficial

to brain health. Don't be afraid to try singing along. If necessary, hide out in the shower while attempting to sing.

10. **Learn:** Study a new language or take a course in an area that interests you. Nowadays, you can choose from countless classes via the internet. If you prefer live instruction, consider signing up for or auditing a course at your local community college.

11. **Cognitive training:** A study by Sherry Willis et al demonstrated that cognitive training for memory, reasoning, and speed of processing resulted in improved cognitive abilities (specific to the training tasks) that continued five years after the initiation of the intervention.[5] Simply put, you can train your brain to improve your ability to reason and recall information. Moreover, practice and training increase the speed with which your brain processes information related to the task you are working on. There are many books and websites that offer opportunities for cognitive training. Card games, crossword puzzles, meditation, chess, learning a new language, and playing a musical instrument are a few ways to perform cognitive training. Enter "cognitive training websites" into your search engine to explore additional opportunities to enhance your cognitive health.

12. **Sleep:** This is so important we'll devote the entire next chapter to it!

13. **Exercise:** Numerous studies demonstrate that regular exercise has a beneficial effect on brain health. For example, a study by Kirk I. Erickson et al found aerobic exercise increases the size of the hippocampus of the brain, leading to improved memory function.[6] If exercising to get in shape isn't enough reason, dust off your sneakers and start moving to aid your memory.

14. **Socialize:** Go out with friends and family, join community groups, and volunteer. One of the numerous benefits of interacting with others is that it stimulates your brain.

15. **Get your hearing checked:** Hearing loss is independently associated with accelerated cognitive decline and cognitive impairment in community-dwelling older adults.[7] The researchers hypothesized if inner ear cells are damaged, they may send a garbled signal to the brain. Since the brain must work harder to decode the message, it may occur at the expense of thinking and memory. Another possibility is that hearing loss leads to social isolation. Rather than asking people to repeat themselves, those with hearing loss may become less engaged, which can lead to impaired cognition. Researchers are currently studying whether hearing aids slow down cognitive decline.

It's a good idea to incorporate the above concepts and ideas into your routine. If this is a particular area of interest to you, there are entire books dedicated to this topic. Be proactive to assist your brain on the path to healthy aging.

Chapter 22

Getting Your ZZZ's: The Importance of a Good Night's Sleep

*T*anya stares up at the ceiling. Once again, sleep eludes her. She finally falls asleep around midnight but then wakes up at 2AM. She's been unable to fall back asleep. It is the same story every night. She tries taking sleeping pills, but they make her feel so groggy the next day. What can she do to get a better night's sleep?

There are numerous health benefits to getting the proper amount of sleep. Sleep provides your body with a chance to repair itself. Getting a good night's rest will help you to concentrate and focus, allowing you to perform better at school and work. If you are fatigued, it's difficult to learn and master new information. With a good night's sleep under your belt, you'll be better able to think more clearly and solve problems. Sleep helps us to process and consolidate our memories from the day. Not only that, but restful sleep may also improve your mood.

Do you need another reason to get your ZZZ's? Getting enough sleep may also improve peoples' sex lives. According to the National Sleep Foundation, up to 26% of those polled said their sex lives were adversely impacted because they were tired.[1] Research is currently being conducted to see if a lack of sleep contributes to low testosterone levels.

Numerous things can get in the way of getting a good night's sleep. Absence of a balance between work, family, and social life can interfere with sleep. Anxiety, worry, and stress also negatively impact sleep. Some people believe sleep is optional, but this is not the case. Furthermore, simply lying in bed doesn't count as sleep.

Pain, both acute and chronic, can make it difficult to sleep. Researchers believe that getting adequate sleep can improve pain levels.

One study found that people who were allowed to sleep for almost two hours longer than usual were less sensitive to pain, as measured by how long it took them to pull their finger away from a heat source.[2] Using the sleep tips listed below can lead to a better night's sleep and hopefully less pain.

It makes sense that getting enough sleep keeps us safer. According to the National Sleep Foundation, people who are sleep-deprived are more likely to get into car accidents.[1] They estimate that each year, one million car accidents in the United States are due to drowsy driving. That equates to an astounding one out of every five crashes. Being drowsy also puts people at risk of getting injured when operating machinery or performing risky activities, like climbing footstools or ladders.

Not getting enough sleep has been linked to diabetes. One study found that people who slept less than six hours per night were 30 percent more likely to develop type II diabetes than those who slept seven hours per night.[3] Lack of sleep is associated with increased inflammation in the body. This may lead to coronary arteries becoming more calcified, which can in turn increase the risk of heart disease. Research shows that people who get less than six hours of sleep per night have a 50 percent higher risk of heart disease than those who get seven or eight hours.[4]

Inadequate sleep can cause weight gain and contribute to obesity. The Nurses' Health Study tracked 68,000 women from 1986 to 2002.[5] They found that women who slept five or six hours gained more weight than those who slept seven or eight. Women who slept only six hours per night were 12 percent more likely to gain 30 pounds over 16 years than women who slept 7 hours per night. Women who slept five or less hours each night were 28 percent more likely.

There are several theories to explain this weight gain. Leptin is a hormone that plays a role in satiety, or the sensation of fullness. Leptin levels drop in people who don't get enough sleep. This causes people to feel hungrier, so they tend to eat more. Even worse, they tend to crave high-fat, calorie-dense foods. In addition, people who are tired may have less energy for exercising or taking the time to cook a healthy meal.

Current research seems to indicate that getting adequate sleep may affect our immune system. Ongoing sleep deprivation may impact the way our immune cells respond. People who get enough sleep may be less likely to catch a cold than those who do not get the recommended amount. In one study, those who got less than seven hours of sleep per night were three times more likely to catch a cold virus than those who slept at least eight hours.[6]

How Much Sleep is Enough?

In March 2015, Max Hirschkowitz, et al published an article regarding sleep duration recommendations in *Sleep Health*, the Journal of the National Sleep Foundation.[7] The National Sleep Foundation's expert panel recommends the following amounts of sleep:

Teenagers (14-17 years)
Recommended Sleep: 8-10 hours
May be Appropriate: 7-11 hours

Young adults (18-25 years)
Recommended Sleep: 9 hours
May be Appropriate: 6-10/11 hours

Adults (26-64 years)
Recommended Sleep: 7-9 hours
May be Appropriate: 6-10 hours

Older adults (greater than 65 years)
Recommended Sleep: 7-8 hours
May be Appropriate: 5/6-9 hours

Steps to a Better Night's Sleep

No one wants to toss and turn at night. Adopting the strategies below may help you get a better night's sleep.

1. Create a comfortable sleeping environment. For many, this means cool (60 to 67 degrees Fahrenheit), dark, and quiet. Consider the use of room-darkening shades as well as fans. Air filters can provide white noise to block out unwanted noise. If you don't want an air filter, consider using a white noise machine.

2. Avoid stimulants: Anything that stimulates your body or makes you more alert can have an adverse effect on sleeping.

   - Avoid all caffeine for at least 6 hours before going to bed. This includes drinks as well as food, such as chocolate.
   - Avoid alcohol for at least 4 hours before bedtime. Alcohol may make you feel drowsy and help you fall asleep, but it won't help you stay asleep. In fact, alcohol may interfere with your sleep later in the night.
   - Avoid decongestant cold medicines at night. They can interfere with your ability to sleep.
   - Don't eat spicy foods for at least 3 hours before bedtime.
   - Avoid nicotine completely or at least before going to bed.
   - Check your list of medications. Are there any side effects that negatively impact sleep? For example, certain cough, cold, and allergy medications can affect sleep.

3. Avoid eating heavy meals a few hours prior to bedtime. Large meals may create discomfort that keeps you awake at night. Similarly, try to avoid going to bed hungry, as this may also create discomfort that makes falling asleep difficult.

4. Avoid evening/nighttime activities that may cause tension or anxiety.

- Avoid watching (or reading) the news before going to bed.
- Avoid paying bills or checking finances before going to bed.
- Avoid arguments prior to bedtime.

5. Plan your sleep.
   - Try to go to sleep and wake up at the same time each day. This helps to reinforce your body's natural sleep-wake cycles.
   - If you don't fall asleep within 30 minutes, get up and do something quiet and non-stimulating. When you feel tired, return to bed, and try going back to sleep.
   - Don't try to "force yourself" to fall asleep, as this may cause anxiety.
   - Avoid afternoon naps. Long naps can interfere with night sleeping. If you nap, limit it to 30 minutes. The exception to this is shift workers, who may need to split their sleep before and after work.

6. Remove potential distractions. This can be a particular problem for those who work the night shift and are trying to sleep during the day.
   - Try using earplugs and eye shades to block out all noise and light.
   - Move the alarm clock away from the bed since it can be a distraction.
   - Silence your cell phone to avoid being disturbed by text alerts. In addition, put it in another room so you won't be tempted to check it if you happen to wake up.
   - Do not watch TV, read, or write in bed. Put away laptops and tablets. The blue light of the screen blocks melatonin from forming, so the brain doesn't get the message that

it's time to sleep. Let your mind and body identify bed with sleeping (and intercourse).

7. Get physically tired.

- Regular exercise (30-45 minutes, 3-5 times per week) may help promote restful sleep. However, avoid vigorous exercise 2-3 hours immediately before bedtime.

8. Give gratitude for 2 to 3 things in your life.

9. Relax.

- Listen to a relaxation program that teaches progressive physical and mental relaxation along with diaphragmatic breathing. Please refer to Chapters 7 and 19 for further information about diaphragmatic breathing.

It's normal to occasionally have a sleepless night. If you try to incorporate some of the above tips into your nighttime routine and still have trouble getting enough ZZZ's, consider consulting your physician. Some people may not get enough sleep due to conditions such as sleep apnea, which requires medical attention.

Chapter 23

Are Anxiety and Depression an Inevitable Part of Aging?

The sun peeks through the blinds of Johanna's bedroom. She rolls over but doesn't get up. What is the point? She feels like nothing good can happen today. As far as she can tell, nothing good ever happens to her. She doesn't have the energy to roll out of bed. Lately, all her bones and joints ache. She isn't hungry for breakfast. In fact, she's dropped ten pounds over the past two months because she's lost her appetite. Would the empty feeling inside her ever go away?

In the above scenario, Johanna is exhibiting some of the common signs and symptoms of depression. Anxiety and depression are NOT a normal, inevitable part of aging. However, both can occur with aging, often due to pre-existing mental health problems or tied to medical conditions. For example, heart attacks, strokes, chronic obstructive pulmonary disease (COPD), Parkinson's disease, cancer, or other ailments can leave people weak and debilitated. This in turn may lead to feelings of sadness, anxiety, or depression. Difficulty getting a good night's sleep can exacerbate the situation.

The Center for Disease Control (CDC) estimates that one to five percent of community-dwelling elderly suffer from major depression.[1] But others may be having symptoms to a lesser degree. The CDC estimates that only 30 percent of older adults who need care for depression actually receive treatment.

The National Institute of Mental Health classifies depression as Major Depression, Dysthymia, and Minor Depression.[2] If a person has Major Depression, it may interfere with sleep, work, appetite, and ability to enjoy life. Dysthymia includes ongoing mild depression that can last two or more years. Minor depression symptoms are less severe and don't last as long as the other types of depression.

Signs of depression in the elderly may be subtle. People who suffer from depression may not complain of feeling sad. Rather, they may report loss of interest in activities, inability to concentrate, generalized aches and pains, or vague intestinal problems.

Anxiety is associated with uneasiness, nervousness, and an apprehensive, unpleasant state. Feeling anxious can be perfectly normal. For example, imagine that you are driving at night and get lost in a seedy-looking neighborhood. Maybe your car breaks down and you left your cell phone at home. It would make sense to feel anxious in this situation. If you decide to go for help and walk down a dark street, anxiety will help you stay alert to danger. Your sense of worry or unease may actually work to keep you safe.

It's normal to feel nervous when you are faced with a big decision. If trying to make choices regarding jobs or relationships, some may feel anxiety. Nervous butterflies would be normal before a big test or exam.

Sometimes, feelings of anxiety occur for unexplained reasons and lead to distress. If these feelings interfere with your daily life, a physician may diagnose you with an anxiety disorder, such as generalized anxiety disorder, panic disorder, or phobias. If you are diagnosed with one of these disorders, your doctor will most likely treat you with medications and counseling (psychotherapy).

The purpose of this chapter is to make you aware that feelings of anxiety and depression are not a normal part of aging. If you or a loved one experiences the signs or symptoms listed above or have thoughts of suicide, consult with your health care practitioner for guidance. If it's a crisis situation, call 911 immediately. Anxiety and depression are both treatable!

Chapter 24

The Power of Prayer

*W*hen *Agnes' phone rings, she isn't prepared for the terrible news. Her friend Martin called to tell her their mutual friend Chantel has suffered a stroke. She's being rushed to the hospital by ambulance. An emergency CT scan of her brain shows a large blood clot in the front part of her brain. They've given her a special medication called tPA, and now she is being rushed into surgery to remove the clot. Martin asks her to start a prayer chain. She says a quick prayer for Chantel's health before calling her friends.*

Have you ever prayed for a friend or family member? Do you go to church? An analysis of 1,500 medical research studies by Harold G. Koenig, M.D., the Director of Spirituality, Theology, and Health at Duke University Medical Center and author of numerous books and research articles, found that prayer can help prevent people from getting sick and can help those who are sick to get better more quickly. In addition, he found that people who pray enjoy better mental and physical health.

Of the 125 studies that looked at the link between regularly attending church and health, 85 studies found regular churchgoers live longer. According to Dr. Koenig, being religious may increase hope and optimism, while lessening anxiety and depression. His analysis of research concluded that those who worship have "stronger immune systems, lower blood pressure, and probably better cardiovascular functioning."

Similarly, a 1998 study by Douglas Oman, PhD and Dwayne Reed, MD, PhD published in the American Journal of Public Health followed 1,931 older residents of Marin County, California over a period of five years.[1] They found that people who attended religious services had significantly lower mortality than those who didn't. Likewise, a study involving 3,968 community-dwelling adults aged 64-101 years residing in the Piedmont of North Carolina demonstrated that older adults, particularly women, who attend religious services at least once a week appear to have a survival advantage over those attending services less frequently. [2]

Believers enjoy other health benefits as well. A study of 3,963 elderly community-dwelling adults studied the relationship between blood pressure and religious activities.[3] Researchers found that religiously active older adults (those who attend religious services and/or study the Bible) tend to have lower blood pressures than those who engage in these activities less frequently.

A 2006 study of 5,300 African Americans by the American Society of Hypertension revealed that those who are involved with religious activities have lower blood pressure than those who don't.[4] They also had lower cortisol levels, which is a biological marker for stress.

There may be benefits for the immune system as well. A study of 1,718 elderly residents of North Carolina (age 65 and older) showed some support for the hypothesis that older adults who frequently attend religious services have healthier immune systems.[5] However, the mechanism of effect was not known.

Praying doesn't just benefit you. It also helps those for whom you are praying. Intercessory prayer is the act of praying to God on behalf of another. Over the last several decades, numerous researchers have attempted to determine the effect of intercessory prayer on various patient outcomes.

A randomized, controlled trial at Saint Luke's Hospital in Kansas City, Missouri looked at the effects of remote, intercessory prayer on the outcomes of 1019 patients admitted to the coronary care unit.[6] Patients were randomly assigned to receive either remote, intercessory prayer (referred to as the "prayer group") or to the "usual care group." The first names of the prayer group were given to Christian intercessors (strangers) who prayed for the patients daily for four weeks. The intercessors were divided into 15 teams of five members each. Each team had a team leader, and team members didn't know each other. Intercessors prayed individually rather than in groups. The Christians included those who identified themselves as non-denominational, Episcopalian, Protestant, and Roman Catholic. The patients in the prayer group weren't aware they were being prayed for. The researchers found that patients in the prayer group had lower overall adverse outcomes as compared to the usual care group, suggesting that prayer could serve as an adjunct to standard medical care.

Dr. Randolph C. Byrd studied cardiac patients from the coronary care unit (CCU) of San Francisco General Hospital to see if intercessory prayer to a Judeo-Christian God effects a patient's medical condition and recovery while in the hospital.[7] Patients were randomly assigned to either a group that received intercessory prayer (192 participants) or did not (201 participants). Patients, staff, and doctors were "blinded," meaning they did not know who was assigned to what group. Intercessors included "born-again" Christians as well as members of several Protestant and Roman Catholic Churches. Each patient in the prayer group was assigned between three and seven intercessors, who were told the patients' first name, diagnosis, general condition, and pertinent updates in their condition. Under the direction of a coordinator, they prayed for the patient daily until he or she was discharged from the hospital. Each intercessor prayed for a rapid recovery and prevention of complications and death. In addition, they could add other prayers that they believed may be beneficial to the patient.

An analysis revealed no statistical differences between the two groups before prayer was initiated. The study found less congestive heart failure, pneumonia, and cardiac arrests in the prayer group. Patients who were prayed for required less diuretic and antibiotic therapy and were less frequently intubated and ventilated. The prayer group had a statistically significant lower severity score based upon the hospital course after entry (p < 0.01). Dr. Byrd points out that prayers by and for the control group could not be controlled, which may have resulted in smaller differences observed between the two groups. His data suggest that "intercessory prayer has a beneficial therapeutic effect in patients admitted to an ICU."

This chapter is by no means designed to be an exhaustive exploration of the scientific evidence in support of the power of prayer. However, it may spark you to reflect on your own involvement in church activities and prayer. Research appears to indicate that being involved in religious activities may benefit your health. Intercessory prayers benefit others. The choice to believe is yours.

Chapter 25

The Healing Power of Forgiveness

Brian hasn't spoken to his brother in twenty-nine years. Not only did Alfred steal his girlfriend, but he married her too. At the time, he vowed he'd never forgive him. But now, he is beginning to waver. Ever since he was diagnosed with pancreatic cancer three weeks ago, he knows it is time to get his affairs in order. Perhaps it is finally time to reach out to Alfred and mend the rift between them.

Holding on to anger and resentment can lead to a multitude of problems, from emotional and psychological distress to outward physical manifestations, like headaches or stomach pain. In short, holding a grudge can make you sick.

What can make you better? Forgiveness. Forgiveness doesn't have to be about the person you are forgiving. It's about helping you to heal so that you can move on with your life and enjoy it again.

Each person reading this book has probably at some time been hurt by the words or actions of a friend, family member, co-worker, or perhaps even a stranger. This can lead to bitterness and perhaps even a determination to "even the score." You may become so wrapped up in your anger that you fail to enjoy the present. It may even place you at odds with your religious and spiritual beliefs.

Forgiveness is more than just accepting an apology. In fact, you can forgive someone even if he or she doesn't apologize. Forgiveness can occur even when reconciliation is not possible, such as in cases in which the person is deceased or unwilling to reconcile. Forgiveness involves letting go of the negative thoughts and anger that you may harbor. It allows you to shed the burden that is weighing you down.

What are the health benefits of forgiveness? Not only can it infuse a sense of peace into your life, but it can also improve your health. There are plenty of reasons to forgive others.

1. **Lower blood pressure and heart rate:** A study in *Psychological Science* demonstrated that unforgiving thoughts tend to raise heart rate and blood pressure, while forgiving thoughts tend to lower them.[1]
2. **Improve your relationships**: If you let go of grudges and exercise forgiveness, you'll have more time and energy to improve current relationships and develop friendships with others.
3. **Decrease stress levels**: Researchers have found that higher levels of lifetime stress and lower levels of forgiveness predicted worse physical and mental health.[2] The authors suggested that forgiving may decrease stress-related disorders.
4. **Lower your pain levels and improve your psychological health**: A study by Carson et al looked at pain levels and forgiveness in patients with chronic low back pain.[3] They found that people with chronic low back pain who express an inability to forgive others tend to have higher levels of pain and psychological distress.
5. **Improve your health and live longer**: The act of forgiveness may result in positive physical health benefits.[4]

Forgiveness can improve your physical, spiritual, and mental health and bring harmony to our lives. It can strengthen your relationship with God and others. In a nutshell, forgiveness brings healing.

The first step to forgiveness is to choose to forgive the person who has hurt you. Remind yourself of the positive value of letting go of your suffering and embracing how forgiveness can improve your life. Say goodbye to your role as victim and don't let your life be defined by pain and hurt. Instead, embrace empathy and understanding.

Chapter 26

It's Time to Volunteer!

Volunteerism is near and dear to my heart. I first started volunteering with my local first aid and rescue squad at age seventeen. I've been answering emergency calls ever since. During the past 35+ years, I've responded to more than 10,000 first aid and fire calls. During my time with the squad, I've been fortunate to witness some truly amazing things. Having the opportunity to help others has been one of the greatest blessings in my life. By giving my time to others, I have found incredible fulfillment.

The benefits of volunteering go beyond making you feel good. The Corporation for National and Community Service performed a review of research regarding the social and health benefits of volunteering.[1] Research shows that long-time volunteers live longer, have less disease, and boast better health. They have lower mortality rates, lower rates of depression, and greater functional ability. Volunteers who devote about 100 hours a year are most likely to enjoy positive health outcomes.

Volunteering has been found to positively impact psychological factors and give one a sense of purpose. Socializing through volunteer work may buffer stress and reduce the risk of disease. Serving others improves life satisfaction. People who volunteer report higher levels of happiness and self-esteem.

As a physical therapist, I treat patients suffering from pain. People with chronic pain report decreased pain intensity and lower levels of disability and depression when serving as peer volunteers for others complaining of chronic pain.[2]

Moreover, individuals who volunteered after suffering a heart attack reported decreased despair and depression, which are two measures that have been linked to increased risk of mortality in patients with coronary artery disease.[3] They also stated they had a greater sense of purpose in their lives.

If that's not enough to convince you to volunteer, consider that people who volunteer may be at a lower risk for developing Alzheimer's disease and dementia.[4] In addition, volunteering may improve brain plasticity. Researchers recruited people at high risk for developing dementia to serve as volunteers in an elementary school.[5] They found evidence for use-dependent brain plasticity, and the volunteers showed improvement in executive brain function.

Volunteering provides a mechanism to help your community while at the same time improving your health. It's a win-win in the quest towards healthy aging.

Chapter 27

The Importance of Relationships

Perhaps one of the most important factors in healthy aging is celebrating our family and friends. Pick up the phone, email, text, or stop by in person. Our relationships with others keep us engaged and connected. According to the Harvard Medical School, satisfying social connections help people to live longer and have fewer health problems.[1] Caring for others decreases stress levels by increasing release of stress-reducing hormones.

In contrast, a lack of strong relationships increases the risk of premature death by 50%. That's the same increase in risk as smoking fifteen cigarettes a day. It's also associated with depression and cognitive decline.

Take a moment to write a list of all the friends and family for which you are thankful. If the list is shorter than you'd like, resolve to meet people and make new friends. As discussed previously, volunteering within the community is a wonderful way to socialize.

Relationships are not just with people. They can be with "fur buddies" too. If you don't have a pet, consider adopting one. There are many senior dogs and cats needing a new home. My family adopted a senior Shih Tzu when he was on the cusp of turning thirteen. He still had lots of pep and energy, and he was a true blessing to our family until he passed at age seventeen.

Dog owners have a lower cardiovascular risk, possibly because dogs provide social support and motivate people to exercise.[2] In addition, pet owners who suffer heart attacks live longer than non-pet owners.[3]

According to the American Heart Association (AHA), owning a pet may lower blood pressure and cholesterol levels.[4]

Owning a pet has been shown to lessen anxiety and depression. They improve our mood and give us a sense of purpose. They fulfill our need for physical touch. Petting a dog triggers the brain to release the hormone oxytocin, which is associated with making people feel good.[5] In addition, it decreases levels of cortisol, a hormone related to stress.

Pets make great conversation starters. Your pooch can help you to socialize and meet others at dog obedience classes, dog parks, or walking in your community. If you can't own a pet, consider volunteering at an animal shelter.

Although owning a pet won't help your adult allergies, studies have shown that children raised in households with pets have a lower risk of developing allergies and asthma. So, if you live with little ones, owning a pet may improve their health.

As an added bonus, dogs need walks. Owning a dog will provide incentive to get off the couch and hit the pavement. According to the AHA, canine owners are 54% more likely to get 30 minutes of daily exercise than those without canine companions.[4] Wouldn't it be wonderful for you and your pet to get in shape together?

In summary, our relationships with other people as well as our pets enhance the quality of our lives. They play an important role in our quest for healthy aging.

Closing Thoughts

Aging is an inevitable part of life. However, we can mitigate the effects by incorporating the ideas and practical strategies described in the previous chapters into our daily routines. Simple lifestyle changes with respect to diet, exercise, spirituality, and mental stimulation can lead to profound changes in our well-being. Healthy aging can be accomplished by focusing on our physical, spiritual, emotional, and cognitive well-being. It's never too late to start!

Appendix A
Bladder Diary

Time of Day	Amount and Type of Fluid/Food Intake	Amount Voided	Amount of Leakage	Was the Urge Present? (Mild, Moderate, Strong)	Activity with leakage/ other comments
12:00AM					
1:00					
2:00					
3:00					
4:00					
5:00					
6:00					
7:00					
8:00					
9:00					
10:00					
11:00					
12:00PM					
1:00					
2:00					
3:00					
4:00					
5:00					
6:00					
7:00					
8:00					
9:00					
10:00					
11:00					

Number of pads used for 24 hour period: _____

Appendix B

Name: _____ Age: _____ Date: _____

Balance Assessment

Do you have a history of falls? Yes/No

If yes, how many falls over what period of time?

_____

Do you use an assistive device? If yes, please specify.

_____

Timed Up and Go (TUG) SCORE: _____seconds

Normative Reference Values by Age:

Age Group (years)	Time (seconds)	95% Confidence Interval (seconds)
60 – 69	8.1	7.1 – 9.0
70 – 79	9.2	8.2 – 10.2
80 – 99	11.3	10.0 – 12.7

Timed Up and Go Cut-off Values Predictive of Falls:

> **14 seconds** associated with high fall risk

> **30 seconds** predictive of needing an assistive device for walking and being dependent (needing total assistance) in ADLs (activities of daily living).

Rhomberg: Eyes Open_____sec. Eyes Closed_____sec.

Interpretation: People should be able to maintain balance with eyes open without swaying for 20-30 seconds.

_____ BASED ON THESE FINDINGS, YOU MAY BENEFIT FROM A REFERRAL TO PHYSICAL THERAPY. PLEASE DISCUSS FINDINGS WITH YOUR DOCTOR.

Notes

Part I: Goodbye Couch Potato:
A Guide to Vascular Health

Chapter 1 Use it or Lose It

1. Kortebein P, Ferrando A, Lombeida J, Wolfe R, Evans WJ. Effect of 10 days of bed rest on skeletal muscle in healthy older adults. JAMA. 2007 Apr 25;297(16):1772-4. doi: 10.1001/jama.297.16.1772-b. PMID: 17456818.

2. Vopat BG, Klinge SA, McClure PK, Fadale PD. The effects of fitness on the aging process. J Am Acad Orthop Surg. 2014 Sep;22(9):576-85. doi: 10.5435/JAAOS-22-09-576. PMID: 25157039.

3. Whelton SP, Chin A, Xin X, He J. Effect of aerobic exercise on blood pressure: a meta-analysis of randomized, controlled trials. Ann Intern Med. 2002 Apr 2;136(7):493-503. doi: 10.7326/0003-4819-136-7-200204020-00006. PMID: 11926784.

4. Durstine JL, Haskell WL. Effects of exercise training on plasma lipids and lipoproteins. Exerc Sport Sci Rev. 1994;22:477-521. PMID: 7925552.

5. Couillard C, Després JP, Lamarche B, Bergeron J, Gagnon J, Leon AS, Rao DC, Skinner JS, Wilmore JH, Bouchard C. Effects of endurance exercise training on plasma HDL cholesterol levels depend on levels of triglycerides: evidence from men of the Health, Risk Factors, Exercise Training and Genetics (HERITAGE) Family Study. Arterioscler Thromb Vasc Biol. 2001 Jul;21(7):1226-32. doi: 10.1161/hq0701.092137. PMID: 11451756.

Chapter 2 Goodbye Couch Potato: Aerobic Activity for Cardiac Health

1. Liu-Ambrose TY, Khan KM, Eng JJ, Heinonen A, McKay HA. Both resistance and agility training increase cortical bone density in 75- to 85-year-old women with low bone mass: a 6-month randomized controlled trial. J Clin Densitom. 2004 Winter;7(4):390-8. doi: 10.1385/jcd:7:4:390. PMID: 15618599.

2. Warburton DE, Nicol CW, Bredin SS. Health benefits of physical activity: the evidence. CMAJ. 2006 Mar 14;174(6):801-9. doi: 10.1503/cmaj.051351. PMID: 16534088; PMCID: PMC1402378.

3. Dunstan DW, Mori TA, Puddey IB, Beilin LJ, Burke V, Morton AR, Stanton KG. The independent and combined effects of aerobic exercise and dietary fish intake on serum lipids and glycemic control in NIDDM. A randomized controlled study. Diabetes Care. 1997 Jun;20(6):913-21. doi: 10.2337/diacare.20.6.913. PMID: 9167099.

4. Holmes MD, Chen WY, Feskanich D, Kroenke CH, Colditz GA. Physical activity and survival after breast cancer diagnosis. JAMA. 2005 May 25;293(20):2479-86. doi: 10.1001/jama.293.20.2479. PMID: 15914748.

5. Haydon AM, Macinnis RJ, English DR, Giles GG. Effect of physical activity and body size on survival after diagnosis with colorectal cancer. Gut. 2006 Jan;55(1):62-7. doi: 10.1136/gut.2005.068189. Epub 2005 Jun 21. PMID: 15972299; PMCID: PMC1856365.

6. Diaz KM, Shimbo D. Physical activity and the prevention of hypertension. Curr Hypertens Rep. 2013 Dec;15(6):659-68. doi: 10.1007/s11906-013-0386-8. PMID: 24052212; PMCID: PMC3901083.

7. Cornelissen VA, Verheyden B, Aubert AE, Fagard RH. Effects of aerobic training intensity on resting, exercise and post-

exercise blood pressure, heart rate and heart-rate variability. J Hum Hypertens. 2010 Mar;24(3):175-82. doi: 10.1038/jhh.2009.51. Epub 2009 Jun 25. PMID: 19554028.

Additional Resources

- Borg GA. Psychophysical bases of perceived exertion. Med Sci Sports Exerc. 1982;14(5):377-81. PMID: 7154893.
- Garber CE, Blissmer B, Deschenes MR, Franklin BA, Lamonte MJ, Lee IM, Nieman DC, Swain DP; American College of Sports Medicine. American College of Sports Medicine position stand. Quantity and quality of exercise for developing and maintaining cardiorespiratory, musculoskeletal, and neuromotor fitness in apparently healthy adults: guidance for prescribing exercise. Med Sci Sports Exerc. 2011 Jul;43(7):1334-59. doi: 10.1249/MSS.0b013e318213fefb. PMID: 21694556.
- Summary of the Surgeon General's report addressing physical activity and health. Nutr Rev. 1996 Sep;54(9):280-4. doi: 10.1111/j.1753-4887.1996.tb03948.x. PMID: 9009669.
- United States Department of Agriculture. "How Many Calories Does Activity Burn?" https://www.choosemyplate.gov/physical-activity-calories-burn

Chapter 4 What You Need to Know About Strokes
1. National Stroke Association. www.stroke.org

Additional Resource

- American Stroke Association (a division of the American Heart Association). https://www.strokeassociation.org/

Chapter 5 Heart Health and Chest Pain

1. Benjamin EJ, Blaha MJ, Chiuve SE, Cushman M, Das SR, Deo R, de Ferranti SD, Floyd J, Fornage M, Gillespie C, Isasi CR, Jiménez MC, Jordan LC, Judd SE, Lackland D, Lichtman JH, Lisabeth L, Liu S, Longenecker CT, Mackey RH, Matsushita K, Mozaffarian D, Mussolino ME, Nasir K, Neumar RW, Palaniappan L, Pandey DK, Thiagarajan RR, Reeves MJ, Ritchey M, Rodriguez CJ, Roth GA, Rosamond WD, Sasson C, Towfighi A, Tsao CW, Turner MB, Virani SS, Voeks JH, Willey JZ, Wilkins JT, Wu JH, Alger HM, Wong SS, Muntner P; American Heart Association Statistics Committee and Stroke Statistics Subcommittee. Heart Disease and Stroke Statistics-2017 Update: A Report From the American Heart Association. Circulation. 2017 Mar 7;135(10):e146-e603. doi: 10.1161/CIR.0000000000000485. Epub 2017 Jan 25. Erratum in: Circulation. 2017 Mar 7;135(10):e646. doi: 10.1161/CIR.0000000000000491. Erratum in: Circulation. 2017 Sep 5;136(10):e196. doi: 10.1161/CIR.0000000000000530. PMID: 28122885; PMCID: PMC5408160.

2. Chris Jagger, "The 25 most common causes of death." Www.medhelp.org, https://www.medhelp.org/general-health/articles/The-25-Most-Common-Causes-of-Death.

3. "Preventable deaths: odds of dying." Www.injuryfacts.org, https://injuryfacts.nsc.org/all-injuries/preventable-death-overview/odds-of-dying.

4. "Number of deaths due to choking in the United States from 1945 to 2017." Www.statistica.com, https://www.statista.com/statistics/527321/deaths-due-to-choking-in-the-us/.

Chapter 6 Keep the Pounds Off: Avoiding Weight Gain

1. Pischon T, Boeing H, Hoffmann K, Bergmann M, Schulze MB, Overvad K, van der Schouw YT, Spencer E, Moons KG, Tjønneland A, Halkjaer J, Jensen MK, Stegger J, Clavel-Chapelon F, Boutron-Ruault MC, Chajes V, Linseisen J, Kaaks R, Trichopoulou A, Trichopoulos D, Bamia C, Sieri S, Palli D, Tumino R, Vineis P, Panico S, Peeters PH, May AM, Bueno-de-Mesquita HB, van Duijnhoven FJ, Hallmans G, Weinehall L, Manjer J, Hedblad B, Lund E, Agudo A, Arriola L, Barricarte A, Navarro C, Martinez C, Quirós JR, Key T, Bingham S, Khaw KT, Boffetta P, Jenab M, Ferrari P, Riboli E. General and abdominal adiposity and risk of death in Europe. N Engl J Med. 2008 Nov 13;359(20):2105-20. doi: 10.1056/NEJMoa0801891. Erratum in: N Engl J Med. 2010 Jun 24;362(25):2433. PMID: 19005195.

2. Estruch R, Ros E, Salas-Salvadó J, Covas MI, Corella D, Arós F, Gómez-Gracia E, Ruiz-Gutiérrez V, Fiol M, Lapetra J, Lamuela-Raventos RM, Serra-Majem L, Pintó X, Basora J, Muñoz MA, Sorlí JV, Martínez JA, Fitó M, Gea A, Hernán MA, Martínez-González MA; PREDIMED Study Investigators. Primary prevention of cardiovascular disease with a Mediterranean diet supplemented with extra-virgin olive oil or nuts. N Engl J Med. 2018 Jun 21;378(25):e34. doi: 10.1056/NEJMoa1800389. Epub 2018 Jun 13. PMID: 29897866.

3. Environmental Working Group. "EWG's 2019 Shopper's Guide to Pesticides in Produce™." EWG's 2019 Shopper's Guide to Pesticides in Produce | Summary. March 20, 2019. https://www.ewg.org/foodnews/summary.php.

4. "Pesticide Data Program." Pesticide Data Program | Agricultural Marketing Service. https://www.ams.usda.gov/datasets/pdp.

Additional Resource

- "Your guide to lowering your blood pressure with DASH." April 2006. Accessed June 16, 2019. https://www.nhlbi.nih.gov/files/docs/public/heart/new_dash.pdf.

Part II: How to Make Your Bladder and Bowels Behave: Say Goodbye to Incontinence, Overactive Bladder, and Constipation

Chapter 7 Healthy "Waterworks": A Guide to Bladder Health, Urinary Incontinence and Urgency/Overactive Bladder, Pelvic Floor Strengthening, and Bladder Retraining

1. The National Association for Continence. http://www.nafc.org.
2. Melville JL, Katon W, Delaney K, Newton K. Urinary incontinence in US women: a population-based study. Arch Intern Med. 2005 Mar 14;165(5):537-42. doi: 10.1001/archinte.165.5.537. PMID: 15767530
3. Minassian VA, Stewart WF, Wood GC. "Urinary incontinence in women." *Obstet Gynecol* 111, no. 2 (2008): 324-331.
4. Waetjen LE, Subak LL, Shen H, Lin F, Wang TH, Vittinghoff E, Brown JS. Stress urinary incontinence surgery in the United States. Obstet Gynecol. 2003 Apr;101(4):671-6. doi: 10.1016/s0029-7844(02)03124-1. PMID: 12681869.
5. Coyne KS, Wein A, Nicholson S, Kvasz M, Chen CI, Milsom I. Economic burden of urgency urinary incontinence in the United States: a systematic review. J Manag Care Pharm. 2014 Feb;20(2):130-40. doi: 10.18553/jmcp.2014.20.2.130. PMID: 24456314; PMCID: PMC10437639.
6. Subak LL, Brown JS, Kraus SR, Brubaker L, Lin F, Richter HE, Bradley CS, Grady D; Diagnostic Aspects of Incontinence

Study Group. The "costs" of urinary incontinence for women. Obstet Gynecol. 2006 Apr;107(4):908-16. doi: 10.1097/01.AOG.0000206213.48334.09. PMID: 16582131; PMCID: PMC1557394.

Additional Resources:

- Chiarelli, Pauline E. *Womens Waterworks: Curing Incontinence.* Wallsend, Australia: George Parry, 2007.
- Gorina Y, Schappert S, Bercovitz A, Elgaddal N, Kramarow E. Prevalence of incontinence among older Americans. Vital Health Stat 3. 2014 Jun;(36):1-33. PMID: 24964267.
- Haylen BT, de Ridder D, Freeman RM, Swift SE, Berghmans B, Lee J, Monga A, Petri E, Rizk DE, Sand PK, Schaer GN; International Urogynecological Association; International Continence Society. An International Urogynecological Association (IUGA)/International Continence Society (ICS) joint report on the terminology for female pelvic floor dysfunction. Neurourol Urodyn. 2010;29(1):4-20. doi: 10.1002/nau.20798. PMID: 19941278.
- Payne CK. Epidemiology, pathophysiology, and evaluation of urinary incontinence and overactive bladder. Urology. 1998 Feb;51(2A Suppl):3-10. doi: 10.1016/s0090-4295(98)90001-2. PMID: 9495728.
- Rodgers AJ, Abraham K. "The importance of monitoring a woman's response to physical therapy intervention in a patient with tension-free vaginal tape-obturator sling failure." *Journal of Women's Health Physical Therapy* 36, no. 1 (April 2012): 4-18. doi:10.1097/jwh.0b013e31824ce539.
- Zinner NR, Koke SC, Viktrup L. Pharmacotherapy for stress urinary incontinence : present and future options. Drugs.

2004;64(14):1503-16. doi: 10.2165/00003495-200464140-00001. PMID: 15233589.

Chapter 8 Don't Let it All Hang Down: Pelvic Organ Prolapse
Additional resource:

- Low pressure fitness website. www.lpf-usa.com

Chapter 9 A Day in the Life of Your Bowels

1. Lewis SJ, Heaton KW. Stool form scale as a useful guide to intestinal transit time. Scand J Gastroenterol. 1997 Sep;32(9):920-4. doi: 10.3109/00365529709011203. PMID: 9299672.

Chapter 10 Constipation 101

1. Garrigues V, Gálvez C, Ortiz V, Ponce M, Nos P, Ponce J. Prevalence of constipation: agreement among several criteria and evaluation of the diagnostic accuracy of qualifying symptoms and self-reported definition in a population-based survey in Spain. Am J Epidemiol. 2004 Mar 1;159(5):520-6. doi: 10.1093/aje/kwh072. PMID: 14977649.
2. "USDA national nutrient database for standard reference, legacy version." US Department of Agriculture, Agricultural Research Service, Nutrient Data Laboratory. April 2018. https://ndb.nal.usda.gov/ndb/nutrients/index

Additional Resource
- "Faux Fiber Versus the Real Thing." @berkeleywellness. December 1, 2011. http://www.berkeleywellness.com/healthy-eating/food/article/faux-fiber-versus-real-thing.

Chapter 11 Staying Hydrated

1. Valtin H. "Drink at least eight glasses of water a day." Really? Is there scientific evidence for "8 x 8"? Am J Physiol Regul Integr Comp Physiol. 2002 Nov;283(5):R993-1004. doi: 10.1152/ajpregu.00365.2002. PMID: 12376390.
2. "Woman dies after being in water-drinking contest." Los Angeles Times/The Associated Press, 14 January 2007.
3. "Georgia teen dies from drinking too much water, gatorade." CBS/The Associated Press, 12 August 2014.

Part III: Keeping Your Framework Healthy: A Guide to Healthy Muscles, Joints, and Bones

Chapter 12 Bone Health: Keeping Your Framework Strong

1. Bone Health and Osteoporosis Foundation https://www.bonehealthandosteoporosis.org/
2. Office of the Surgeon General (US). Bone Health and Osteoporosis: A Report of the Surgeon General. Rockville (MD): Office of the Surgeon General (US); 2004. PMID: 20945569.
3. Burge R, Dawson-Hughes B, Solomon DH, Wong JB, King A, Tosteson A. Incidence and economic burden of osteoporosis-related fractures in the United States, 2005-2025. J Bone Miner Res. 2007 Mar;22(3):465-75. doi: 10.1359/jbmr.061113. PMID: 17144789.
4. Hartley GW, Roach KE, Nithman RW, Betz SR, Lindsey C, Fuchs RK, Avin KG. Physical Therapist Management of Patients With Suspected or Confirmed Osteoporosis: A Clinical Practice Guideline From the Academy of Geriatric Physical Therapy. J Geriatr Phys Ther. 2022 Apr-Jun 01;44(2):80. doi: 10.1519/JPT.0000000000000357. PMID: 35384942.

Andrea Jo Rodgers

Additional Resources

- Warburton DE, Nicol CW, Bredin SS. Health benefits of physical activity: the evidence. CMAJ. 2006 Mar 14;174(6):801-9. doi: 10.1503/cmaj.051351. PMID: 16534088; PMCID: PMC1402378.
- Bérard, A., G. Bravo, and P. Gauthier. "Meta-analysis of the effectiveness of physical activity for the prevention of bone loss in postmenopausal women." *Osteoporosis International* 7, no. 4 (1997): 331-37. doi:10.1007/bf01623773.
- Bonaiuti D, Shea B, Iovine R, Negrini S, Robinson V, Kemper HC, Wells G, Tugwell P, Cranney A. Exercise for preventing and treating osteoporosis in postmenopausal women. Cochrane Database Syst Rev. 2002;(3):CD000333. doi: 10.1002/14651858.CD000333. Update in: Cochrane Database Syst Rev. 2011 Jul 06;(7):CD000333. doi: 10.1002/14651858.CD000333.pub2. PMID: 12137611.
- "Calcium and Vitamin D." Bone Health and Osteoporosis Foundation. Accessed Apr 4, 2024. https://www.bonehealthandosteoporosis.org/patients/treatment/calciumvitamin-d/
- Kelley GA. Exercise and regional bone mineral density in postmenopausal women: a meta-analytic review of randomized trials. Am J Phys Med Rehabil. 1998 Jan-Feb;77(1):76-87. PMID: 9482383.
- "Calcium content of common foods." Calcium Content of Common Foods | International Osteoporosis Foundation. https://www.iofbonehealth.org/osteoporosis-musculoskeletal-disorders/osteoporosis/prevention/calcium/
- Kemmler W, Shojaa M, Kohl M, von Stengel S. Effects of different types of exercise on bone mineral density in

257

postmenopausal women: a systematic review and meta-analysis. Calcif Tissue Int. 2020 Nov;107(5):409-439. doi: 10.1007/s00223-020-00744-w. Epub 2020 Aug 12. PMID: 32785775; PMCID: PMC7546993.

- Liu-Ambrose TY, Khan KM, Eng JJ, Heinonen A, McKay HA. Both resistance and agility training increase cortical bone density in 75- to 85-year-old women with low bone mass: a 6-month randomized controlled trial. J Clin Densitom. 2004 Winter;7(4):390-8. doi: 10.1385/jcd:7:4:390. PMID: 15618599.

- Snow CM, Shaw JM, Winters KM, Witzke KA. Long-term exercise using weighted vests prevents hip bone loss in postmenopausal women. J Gerontol A Biol Sci Med Sci. 2000 Sep;55(9):M489-91. doi: 10.1093/gerona/55.9.m489. PMID: 10995045. Christine M.

- Wolff I, van Croonenborg JJ, Kemper HC, Kostense PJ, Twisk JW. The effect of exercise training programs on bone mass: a meta-analysis of published controlled trials in pre- and postmenopausal women. Osteoporos Int. 1999;9(1):1-12. doi: 10.1007/s001980050109. PMID: 10367023.

Chapter 13

1. Shrier I. Stretching before exercise does not reduce the risk of local muscle injury: a critical review of the clinical and basic science literature. Clin J Sport Med 1999;9: 221-227.

Chapter 14 Back Basics for a Healthy Spine

1. "Low back pain facts sheet." National Institute for Neurological Disorders and Stroke. https://www.ninds.nih.gov/Disorders/Patient-Caregiver-Education/Fact-Sheets/Low-Back-Pain-Fact-Sheet

Chapter 16 Avoiding Skin Cancer and Keeping Your Youthful Appearance

1. Stern RS. Prevalence of a history of skin cancer in 2007: results of an incidence-based model. Arch Dermatol. 2010 Mar;146(3):279-82. doi: 10.1001/archdermatol.2010.4. PMID: 20231498.
2. The Lewin Group, Inc. "The burden of skin diseases 2005." Prepared for the Society for Investigative Dermatology, Cleveland, OH, and the American Academy of Dermatology Assn., Washington, DC, 2005.
3. "Cancer facts and figures 2018." Atlanta: American Cancer Society, 2018. https://www.cancer.org/content/dam/cancer-org/research/cancer-facts-and-statistics/annual-cancer-facts-and-figures/2018/cancer-facts-and-figures-2018.pdf.
4. Pfahlberg A, Kölmel KF, Gefeller O; Febim Study Group. Timing of excessive ultraviolet radiation and melanoma: epidemiology does not support the existence of a critical period of high susceptibility to solar ultraviolet radiation- induced melanoma. Br J Dermatol. 2001 Mar;144(3):471-5. doi: 10.1046/j.1365-2133.2001.04070.x. PMID: 11260001.
5. Skin Cancer Foundation. https://www.skincancer.org
6. American Academy of Dermatology. https://www.aad.org
7. Wehner MR, Chren MM, Nameth D, Choudhry A, Gaskins M, Nead KT, Boscardin WJ, Linos E. International prevalence of indoor tanning: a systematic review and meta-analysis. JAMA Dermatol. 2014 Apr;150(4):390-400. doi: 10.1001/jamadermatol.2013.6896. Erratum in: JAMA Dermatol. 2014 May;150(5):577. PMID: 24477278; PMCID: PMC4117411.
8. "Food news." Environmental Working Group (EWG), 2019. https://www.ewg.org/foodnews/

9. "Skin deep cosmetic safety database." Environmental Working Group (EWG), 2019. https://www.ewg.org/skindeep/

10. "EWG's guide to healthy cleaning." Environmental Working Group (EWG), 2019. https://www.ewg.org/guides/cleaners.

11. B. C. Wolverton. *How to Grow Fresh Air: 50 House Plants that Purify Your Home or Office*, New York: NY: Penguin Books, 1 April 1997.

Chapter 18 Strategies to Improve Balance and Prevent Falls

1. "Falls prevention facts." The National Council on Aging (NCOA). June 04, 2018. https://www.ncoa.org/news/resources-for-reporters/get-the-facts/falls-prevention-facts/.

Chapter 19 The Effects of Stress and Coping Strategies

1. The American Psychological Association Report on Stress (2017). www.apa.org

2. The American Psychological Association Report on Stress (2013). www.apa.org

Chapter 20 Understanding the Basics of Cancer

1. "Cancer prevalence: how many people have cancer?" https://www.cancer.org/cancer/cancer-basics/cancer-prevalence.html.

Chapter 21 Keep Your Brain Active

1. "Alzheimer's disease and dementia." The Alzheimer's Association. https://alz.org/.

2. Luciano M, Corley J, Cox SR, Valdés Hernández MC, Craig LC, Dickie DA, Karama S, McNeill GM, Bastin ME, Wardlaw JM, Deary IJ. Mediterranean-type diet and brain structural change

from 73 to 76 years in a Scottish cohort. Neurology. 2017 Jan 31;88(5):449-455. doi: 10.1212/WNL.0000000000003559. Epub 2017 Jan 4. PMID: 28053008; PMCID: PMC5278943.

3. Xu WL, Atti AR, Gatz M, Pedersen NL, Johansson B, Fratiglioni L. Midlife overweight and obesity increase late-life dementia risk: a population-based twin study. Neurology. 2011 May 3;76(18):1568-74. doi: 10.1212/WNL.0b013e3182190d09. PMID: 21536637; PMCID: PMC3100125.

4. Wilson RS, Barnes LL, Aggarwal NT, Boyle PA, Hebert LE, Mendes de Leon CF,   Evans DA. "Cognitive activity and the cognitive morbidity of Alzheimer's disease." *Neurology,* 75, no. 11, (2010): 990-96.

5. Willis SL, Tennstedt SL, Marsiske M, Ball K, Elias J, Koepke KM, Morris JN, Rebok GW, Unverzagt FW, Stoddard AM, Wright E; ACTIVE Study Group. Long-term effects of cognitive training on everyday functional outcomes in older adults. JAMA. 2006 Dec 20;296(23):2805-14. doi: 10.1001/jama.296.23.2805. PMID: 17179457; PMCID: PMC2910591.

6. Erickson KI, Voss MW, Prakash RS, Basak C, Szabo A, Chaddock L, Kim JS, Heo S, Alves H, White SM, Wojcicki TR, Mailey E, Vieira VJ, Martin SA, Pence BD, Woods JA, McAuley E, Kramer AF. Exercise training increases size of hippocampus and improves memory. Proc Natl Acad Sci U S A. 2011 Feb 15;108(7):3017-22. doi: 10.1073/pnas.1015950108. Epub 2011 Jan 31. PMID: 21282661; PMCID: PMC3041121.

7. Lin FR, Yaffe K, Xia J, Xue QL, Harris TB, Purchase-Helzner E, Satterfield S, Ayonayon HN, Ferrucci L, Simonsick EM; Health ABC Study Group. Hearing loss and cognitive decline in older adults. JAMA Intern Med. 2013 Feb 25;173(4):293-9. doi: 10.1001/jamainternmed.2013.1868. PMID: 23337978; PMCID: PMC3869227.

Additional Resource

- Williams JW, Plassman BL, Burke J, Holsinger T, and Benjamin S. "Preventing Alzheimer's disease and cognitive decline." *Evidence Report/Technology Assessment No. 193.* (Prepared by the Duke Evidence-based Practice Center under Contract No. HHSA 290-2007-10066-I.) AHRQ Publication No. 10-E005. Rockville, MD: Agency for Healthcare Research and Quality, April 2010.
- Sparrman, Bonnie. *60 Ways to Keep Your Brain Sharp: Helpful Habits for a Clear Mind and a Great Memory.* Harvest House Publishers, 2018.

Chapter 22 Getting Your ZZZ's: The Importance of a Good Night's Sleep

1. National Sleep Foundation. www.drowsydriving.org
2. Roehrs TA, Harris E, Randall S, Roth T. Pain sensitivity and recovery from mild chronic sleep loss. Sleep. 2012 Dec 1;35(12):1667-72. doi: 10.5665/sleep.2240. PMID: 23204609; PMCID: PMC3490359.
3. Holliday EG, Magee CA, Kritharides L, Banks E, Attia J. Short sleep duration is associated with risk of future diabetes but not cardiovascular disease: a prospective study and meta-analysis. PLoS One. 2013 Nov 25;8(11):e82305. doi: 10.1371/journal.pone.0082305. PMID: 24282622; PMCID: PMC3840027.
4. Cappuccio FP, Cooper D, D'Elia L, Strazzullo P, Miller MA. Sleep duration predicts cardiovascular outcomes: a systematic review and meta-analysis of prospective studies. Eur Heart J. 2011 Jun;32(12):1484-92. doi: 10.1093/eurheartj/ehr007. Epub 2011 Feb 7. PMID: 21300732.

5.   Patel, SR, Malhotra A, White DP, Gottlieb DJ, Hu FB (2006). Association between reduced sleep and weight gain in women. *Am J Epidemiol* 164, no. 10 (2006): 947-54. doi:10.1093/aje/kwj280.

6.   Cohen S, Doyle WJ, Alper CM, Janicki-Deverts D, Turner RB. Sleep habits and susceptibility to the common cold. Arch Intern Med. 2009 Jan 12;169(1):62-7. doi: 10.1001/archinternmed.2008.505. PMID: 19139325; PMCID: PMC2629403.

7.   Hirshkowitz M, Whiton K, Albert SM, Alessi C, Bruni O, DonCarlos L, Hazen N, Herman J, Katz ES, Kheirandish-Gozal L, Neubauer DN, O'Donnell AE, Ohayon M, Peever J, Rawding R, Sachdeva RC, Setters B, Vitiello MV, Ware JC, Adams Hillard PJ. National Sleep Foundation's sleep time duration recommendations: methodology and results summary. Sleep Health. 2015 Mar;1(1):40-43. doi: 10.1016/j.sleh.2014.12.010. Epub 2015 Jan 8. PMID: 29073412.

Chapter 23 Are Anxiety and Depression an Inevitable Part of Aging?

1.   "Mental health." Centers for Disease Control and Prevention. https://www.cdc.gov/mentalhealth/.

2.   National Institute of Mental Health NIH). https://www.nimh.nih.gov/index.shtml

Chapter 24: The Power of Prayer

1.   Oman D, Reed D. Religion, and mortality among the community-dwelling elderly. Am J Public Health. 1998 Oct;88(10):1469-75. doi: 10.2105/ajph.88.10.1469. PMID: 9772846; PMCID: PMC1508463.

2. Koenig HG, Hays JC, Larson DB, George LK, Cohen HJ, McCullough ME, Meador KG, Blazer DG. Does religious attendance prolong survival? A six-year follow-up study of 3,968 older adults. J Gerontol A Biol Sci Med Sci. 1999 Jul;54(7):M370-6. doi: 10.1093/gerona/54.7.m370. PMID: 10462170.

3. Koenig HG, George LK, Hays JC, Larson DB, Cohen HJ, Blazer DG. The relationship between religious activities and blood pressure in older adults. Int J Psychiatry Med. 1998;28(2):189-213. doi: 10.2190/75JM-J234-5JKN-4DQD. PMID: 9724889.

4. American Society of Hypertension 21st Annual Scientific Meeting, New York City, May 16-20, 2006. Sharon Wyatt, RN, PhD, University of Mississippi Medical Center, Jackson. Thomas D. Giles, MD, professor of medicine, Louisiana State University School of Medicine, New Orleans; and president, American Society of Hypertension.

5. Koenig HG, Cohen HJ, George LK, Hays JC, Larson DB, Blazer DG. Attendance at religious services, interleukin-6, and other biological parameters of immune function in older adults. Int J Psychiatry Med. 1997;27(3):233-50. doi: 10.2190/40NF-Q9Y2-0GG7-4WH6. PMID: 9565726.

6. Harris WS, Gowda M, Kolb JW, Strychacz CP, Vacek JL, Jones PG, Forker A, O'Keefe JH, McCallister BD. A randomized, controlled trial of the effects of remote, intercessory prayer on outcomes in patients admitted to the coronary care unit. Arch Intern Med. 1999 Oct 25;159(19):2273-8. doi: 10.1001/archinte.159.19.2273. Erratum in: Arch Intern Med 2000 Jun 26;160(12):1878. PMID: 10547166.

7. Byrd RC. Positive therapeutic effects of intercessory prayer in a coronary care unit population. South Med J. 1988 Jul;81(7):826-9. doi: 10.1097/00007611-198807000-00005. PMID: 3393937.

Chapter 25 The Healing Power of Forgiveness

1. vanOyen Witvliet C, Ludwig TE, Vander Laan KL. Granting forgiveness or harboring grudges: implications for emotion, physiology, and health. Psychol Sci. 2001 Mar;12(2):117-23. doi: 10.1111/1467-9280.00320. PMID: 11340919.
2. Toussaint L, Shields GS, Dorn G, Slavich GM. Effects of lifetime stress exposure on mental and physical health in young adulthood: How stress degrades and forgiveness protects health. J Health Psychol. 2016 Jun;21(6):1004-14. doi: 10.1177/1359105314544132. Epub 2014 Aug 19. PMID: 25139892; PMCID: PMC4363296.
3. Carson JW, Keefe FJ, Goli V, Fras AM, Lynch TR, Thorp SR, Buechler JL. Forgiveness and chronic low back pain: a preliminary study examining the relationship of forgiveness to pain, anger, and psychological distress. J Pain. 2005 Feb;6(2):84-91. doi: 10.1016/j.jpain.2004.10.012. PMID: 15694874.
4. Toussaint LL, Owen AD, Cheadle A. Forgive to live: forgiveness, health, and longevity. J Behav Med. 2012 Aug;35(4):375-86. doi: 10.1007/s10865-011-9362-4. Epub 2011 Jun 25. PMID: 21706213.

Chapter 26 It's Time to Volunteer!

1. Grimm Jr. R, Spring K, Dietz N. Health Benefits of Volunteering: A Review of Recent Research, New York, NY: Corporation for National and Community Service, April 2007.
2. Arnstein P, Vidal M, Wells-Federman C, Morgan B, Caudill M. From chronic pain patient to peer: benefits and risks of volunteering. Pain Manag Nurs. 2002 Sep;3(3):94-103. doi: 10.1053/jpmn.2002.126069. PMID: 12198640.
3. Sullivan GB, Sullivan MJ. Promoting wellness in cardiac rehabilitation: exploring the role of altruism. J Cardiovasc Nurs.

1997 Apr;11(3):43-52. doi: 10.1097/00005082-199704000-00005. PMID: 9095453.

4. Griep Y, Hanson LM, Vantilborgh T, Janssens L, Jones SK, Hyde M. Can volunteering in later life reduce the risk of dementia? A 5-year longitudinal study among volunteering and non-volunteering retired seniors. PLoS One. 2017 Mar 16;12(3):e0173885. doi: 10.1371/journal.pone.0173885. PMID: 28301554; PMCID: PMC5354395.

5. Carlson MC, Erickson KI, Kramer AF, Voss MW, Bolea N, Mielke M, McGill S, Rebok GW, Seeman T, Fried LP. Evidence for neurocognitive plasticity in at-risk older adults: the experience corps program. J Gerontol A Biol Sci Med Sci. 2009 Dec;64(12):1275-82. doi: 10.1093/gerona/glp117. Epub 2009 Aug 19. PMID: 19692672; PMCID: PMC2781785.

Chapter 27 The Importance of Relationships

1. Harvard Health Publishing. "The health benefits of strong relationships." Harvard Health, December 2010. https://www.health.harvard.edu/newsletter_article/the-health-benefits-of-strong-relationships.

2. Mubanga M, Byberg L, Nowak C, Egenvall A, Magnusson PK, Ingelsson E, Fall T. Dog ownership and the risk of cardiovascular disease and death - a nationwide cohort study. Sci Rep. 2017 Nov 17;7(1):15821. doi: 10.1038/s41598-017-16118-6. PMID: 29150678; PMCID: PMC5693989.

3. Friedmann E, Thomas SA. Pet ownership, social support, and one-year survival after acute myocardial infarction in the Cardiac Arrhythmia Suppression Trial (CAST). Am J Cardiol. 1995 Dec 15;76(17):1213-7. doi: 10.1016/s0002-9149(99)80343-9. PMID: 7502998.

4. American Heart Association. https://www.heart.org/

5. Petersson M, Uvnäs-Moberg K, Nilsson A, Gustafson LL, Hydbring-Sandberg E, Handlin L. Oxytocin and Cortisol Levels in Dog Owners and Their Dogs Are Associated with Behavioral Patterns: An Exploratory Study. Front Psychol. 2017 Oct 13;8:1796. doi: 10.3389/fpsyg.2017.01796. PMID: 29081760; PMCID: PMC5645535.

About The Author

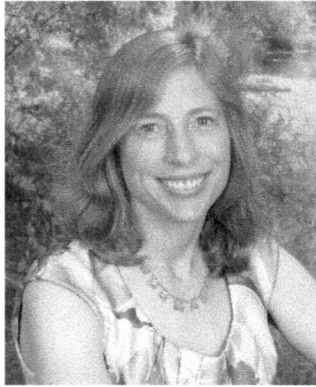

Andrea Jo Rodgers holds a clinical doctorate in physical therapy and has worked as a physical therapist for 30 years. She is CAPP-certified in pelvic health by the American Physical Therapy Association, a nationally certified lymphedema therapist, a PORi-certified oncology rehabilitation therapist, and a low pressure fitness instructor. She also specializes in orthopedics, osteoporosis, and amyotrophic lateral sclerosis (ALS). Writing is one of her passions, and she is the award-winning author of numerous inspirational books. She has served as a volunteer emergency medical technician on her town's rescue squad for 38 years and has responded to 10,000 first aid and fire calls. She enjoys reading, day trips, and savoring a cup of green tea. She lives with her family on the east coast.

Books By Andrea Jo Rodgers

Saving Mount Rushmore

Saving the Statue of Liberty

At Heaven's Edge: True Stories of Faith and Rescue

On Heaven's Doorstep: God's Help in Times of Crisis-True Stories
from a First Responder

Help From Heaven: True Stories of Rescues, Miracles, and Answered
Prayers

Heaven-Sent Miracles & Rescues: True Stories from a First Responder

Heavenly Rescues & Answered Prayers: True Stories of Faith and
Miracles from a First Responder

A Practical Guide to Healthy Aging: Strategies to Achieve Physical and
Mental Health